How to Cure Almost Any Cancer at Home for $5.15 A Day

By Bill Henderson with Andrew Scholberg

How to Cure Almost Any Cancer at Home for $5.15 a Day

By Bill Henderson with Andrew Scholberg

Published by Online Publishing & Marketing, LLC

A Publication from *Cancer Defeated!*

IMPORTANT CAUTION:

By reading this special report you are demonstrating an interest in maintaining good and vigorous health.

This report suggests ways you can do that, but — as with anything in medicine — there are no guarantees.

You must check with private, professional medical advisors to assess whether the suggestions in this report are appropriate for you. And please note, the contents of this report may be considered controversial by the medical community at large.

The author, editors and publishers of this report are not doctors or professional health caregivers. The information in this report is not meant to replace the attention or advice of physicians or other healthcare professionals. Nothing contained in this report is meant to constitute personal medical advice for any particular individual. Every reader who wishes to begin any dietary, drug, exercise or other lifestyle changes intended to treat a specific disease or health condition should first get the advice of a qualified health care professional, or accept full responsibility if he or she decides not to do that.

No alternative OR mainstream cancer treatment can boast a one hundred percent record of success. Far from it. There is ALWAYS some risk involved in any cancer treatment. The author, editors, and publishers of this report are not responsible for any adverse effects or results from the use of any of the suggestions, preparations or procedures described in this report. As with any medical treatment, results of the treatments described in this report will vary from one person to another.

PLEASE DO NOT USE THIS REPORT IF YOU ARE NOT WILLING TO ASSUME THE RISK.

The author reports here the results of a vast array of treatments and research as well as the personal experiences of individual patients, healthcare professionals and caregivers. In most cases the author was not present himself to witness the events described but relied in good faith on the accounts of the people who were.

ISBN 978-1-61539-952-9

© Copyright 2012 by Online Publishing & Marketing, LLC, P.O. Box 1076, Lexington, VA 24450
All rights reserved. No part of this publication may be reproduced, stored in a retrieval system, or transmitted in any form or by any means, electronic, mechanical, photocopying, recording or otherwise, without the prior written permission of the copyright owner.

Printed in the United States of America

About the Authors

Bill Henderson is a retired Air Force Colonel and retired business owner. In November 1990, his late wife, Marjorie, began her four-year bout with ovarian cancer. She died on November 1, 1994. Her many operations, chemotherapy treatments and intense pain made her wish often in her last two years for a quick death, or "transition," as she called it.

After watching her suffering, it was hard for Bill to believe that millions of people each year had to endure that same torture. He now believes the treatment she received, *not the cancer itself,* was the cause of her death.

He has read widely in the ensuing years, searching for alternative cancer treatments. His first book, *Cure Your Cancer,* was the result of his search. First published as an e-book in November of 2000, it quickly became popular all over the world, thanks to the power of the Internet. Readers in 59 countries have used the information in that book to become cancer-free. It was so successful, Bill Henderson published it as a paperback and hard cover book in July 2003. He soon followed with his second book, *Cancer-Free,* published as an e-book and paperback in November of 2004, which is now in its fourth edition, published in November 2011.

He has built a vast network of cancer doctors, nurses, cancer survivors and cancer crusaders. He publishes an Internet newsletter with a readership of over 34,000 in 88 countries. His radio show "How to Live Cancer-Free" attracts 75,000 listeners every week on www.WebTalkRadio.net.

Andrew Scholberg is a freelance writer living in Chicago, Illinois, as well as a devotee of alternative medicine. He's the author of the special report *German Cancer Breakthrough* and the co-author, along with cancer activist Frank Cousineau, of the special reports *Adios, Cancer!* and *Cancer Breakthrough USA!* He is also the co-author, along with Ty Bollinger, of the special report *The 31-Day Home Cancer Cure.* He was the defendant in a landmark First Amendment case before the Supreme Court. In his spare time, Andrew is an adventurous outdoorsman.

Table Of Contents

Chapter One
The day that changed my life forever..1

Chapter Two
The little-known link between root canals and cancer 7

Chapter Three
A hidden cause of many cancers: emotional shock or stress............ 11

Chapter Four
Change your eating plan and *save your life!* 14

Chapter Five
What I would do if *I* had cancer:
My simple seven-point program for *any* type of cancer 23

Chapter Six
Should you go to an alternative cancer clinic? 33

Chapter Seven
What is a cancer coach, and do you need one? 44

Chapter One
The day that changed my life forever

My life changed on November 1, 1994. On that day, my beloved first wife died following years of cancer treatments. These treatments were so harsh that they destroyed what Marge most needed to beat cancer: her immune system.

My wife's cancer treatments were torture. She had one surgery after another — but to no avail. And the radiation and endless rounds of chemotherapy made her so sick she felt like hell. She was in pain. She yearned for a "transition."

She wanted to die, and she did.

After Marge's death, I thought long and hard about the misery the American cancer treatment industry had put her through. I couldn't shake the thought that there *had* to be a better way — a gentler, more effective way to get rid of cancer.

I had a hunch that the cancer didn't kill Marge. I suspected that the cancer *treatments* killed her — the very treatments most Americans take for granted: surgery, radiation, and chemotherapy. I now call these three treatments "cut, burn, poison."

And so I followed up my hunch with a massive research effort to find the truth. It turned into a full-time quest for a better way to treat cancer — a quest that consumes me to this very day.

And now, having studied just about everything I could find about cancer, I'm absolutely 100 percent convinced that my hunch was correct: the harsh "medical" treatments killed my wife — not the cancer.

For the last 13 years, a day hasn't gone by when I haven't been working on alternative cancer treatments: researching, reading, studying, and helping patients beat cancer with gentle, effective, non-toxic treatments.

During that time I've found *several* effective ways to get rid of cancer. And I've helped thousands of people all over the world beat the death sentences their doctors had given them.

Typically, an American doctor will tell a stage-3 or stage-4 cancer patient something like this: "You have three to six months to live." But that doesn't mean anything, unless the patient believes it. Through my best-selling book *Cancer-Free: Your Guide to Gentle, Non-toxic Healing* I've helped countless "terminal" and "hopeless" cancer patients prove those doctors wrong.

For example, one of my clients is a wonderful young lady from San Diego who was struggling with breast cancer. She told me her oncologist was even more aggressive than a used car salesman, relentlessly pressuring her to undergo his harsh treatments. Instead, she got rid of her cancer by using my natural treatment plan.

As a cancer coach, I've personally worked with *thousands* of patients, helping them overcome even the most difficult cases of "terminal" cancer. In fact, it's normal to melt cancer away in a matter of weeks when you follow my method. And it's not expensive, either.

The American cancer treatment industry will charge you about $1,200,000 to die of cancer. Granted, many people have insurance that will pay for it, but who has that kind of

money just lying around?

By contrast, the program I recommend can help any American — even the uninsured — to beat cancer for only $5.15 a day. Just about everybody can afford that.

No doctor should give a cancer patient a death sentence, saying, "You have three to six months to live." No doctor can predict the future, though they routinely make such predictions. I know many patients who proved their doctors wrong by taking their health into their own hands.

Nor should any doctor tell a cancer patient that "nothing more can be done." This can *devastate* the patient. And it's totally false because no doctor can know *everything*. Instead, doctors should say, "I don't know of anything more that can be done." That would be more honest.

I've spoken to over 3,500 cancer victims in 63 countries in the last few years. You might find this hard to believe, but not one of them had heard anything about the *cause* of cancer from their doctors. That's right. Not even one.

Why don't doctors tell their patients the cause of cancer? Maybe it's because they don't know what causes it.

When I first talk to patients, they're scared. But when I explain the three main causes of cancer, and when they see eye to eye with me about those causes, they begin to see a way to reverse the cancer. They see a bright ray of hope.

What, then, are the causes of cancer? During my thousands of hours of research, I've identified three principal causes.

Hidden culprit No. 1 exposed: Root canals and other jaw problems

You might be surprised to know that root canals and other jaw problems can cause cancer. Although you might not link cancer with oral health, it's a well-known fact that oral health affects much more than just your mouth. Inflammation in the gums or toxic pockets in the jaw can tear the immune system to shreds.

I've found that about 70 to 80 percent of the cancer victims I coach have root canals. And, in my opinion, the evidence is overwhelming that these root canals are linked to the cancer. When a root canal is the cause of someone's cancer, then obviously it would do no good to focus only on getting rid of the cancer. The cancer would simply come back. That's what happens when you treat the symptom while ignoring the cause.

But when root canals are the culprit and cancer patients get the root canals removed, the patients just about always get better quickly — almost 100 percent. And I can make that statement based on my vast experience with more than 3,500 cancer sufferers.

In the next chapter I'm going to tell you how to find someone who's competent to evaluate your oral health if you're concerned that a root canal or an improperly extracted wisdom tooth could be the hidden cause of cancer or other health problems.

Hidden culprit No. 2: Unresolved emotional stress

It might also surprise you to know that unresolved emotional stress can cause cancer.

Now, I disagree with those who claim that 90 percent or more of cancer cases are linked to emotional issues. But I'm convinced that more than half of cancer cases stem from some kind of emotional shock, trauma, or issue.

When someone gets cancer, it's worth asking whether a jarring event has taken place in the patient's life within the last year

or so. Has he or she suffered the death of a loved one, the loss of a job, a divorce, or some other stress? Having talked to thousands of cancer victims, I'd estimate that some kind of emotionally jarring event is a factor in well over half of cancer cases. And in chapter three I'm going to tell you how to resolve these problems quickly and easily. It's totally unnecessary to spend years on a psychotherapist's couch.

Culprit No. 3: The American Diet

As you probably know, one of the biggest causes of cancer is our diet, our food, what we put into our mouths, what we buy at the grocery store. When a lifetime of bad eating is combined with faulty dental work, you're likely to get cancer. And if you throw in an emotional trauma like a death in the family, you've practically got a target on your back for this dreaded disease.

The typical American diet is unhealthy and has few nutrients. It gives cancer everything it could possibly want: lots of refined sugar, high fructose corn syrup, preservatives, artificial chemicals, added hormones, and hydrogenated oil.

In chapter four I'm going to give you an eating plan that will keep you out of trouble.

The three causes I've just mentioned — root canals, emotional issues, and the typical American diet — pretty well nail the principal causes of cancer. But there are some other causes. Of course, it's well known that smoking or chewing tobacco causes cancer. Some other causes include environmental toxins, radiation, and vaccinations.

Incredible as it sounds, many vaccinations contain known poisons such as mercury and even formaldehyde. Is this insane, or what? How can injecting these poisons possibly be safe?

The four secrets of treating and beating cancer

Because cancer comes from within the patient's body, whatever treatment the patient selects must *address four factors*:

1) Cancer treatment must strengthen the immune system. Cancer cells are normally "no big deal." Everybody produces cancer cells every day. But a strong and healthy immune system can mop up cancer cells faster than our bodies can produce them. When cancer runs out of control, you can be sure that the immune system has become too weak to kill off the multiplying cancer cells.

2) Cancer treatment must increase the oxygenation of the cells. Cancer cells are anaerobic; they need *sugar* to thrive and multiply. They *hate* oxygen. Cancer cells react to oxygenation the way a vampire would react to broad daylight. And when healthy cells get more oxygen, they produce more energy. Your health becomes more vibrant.

3) Cancer treatment must detoxify the body. Toxins put a heavy stress on the immune system. Getting rid of the toxins helps the body get back into a state of vibrant health. In chapter four I'm going to give you an eating plan that won't just nourish you but will also detoxify you.

4) Cancer treatment must change the body chemistry from acidic to alkaline. Cancer and other diseases thrive in an acidic body. But you can easily change your body chemistry. And when your body becomes alkaline, cancer gets the message that it's no longer welcome and will no longer be tolerated. The program I recommend promotes an alkaline state.

Let me emphasize that *any* treatment plan must address *all four* of these factors! When I get this point across to my cancer-coaching clients, they begin to evaluate in their own minds how chemo and radiation would fit

into those four factors. They don't fit! In fact, chemo and radiation can make all four factors worse!

I've never had cancer. But as a result of my relentless quest for information about the most effective cancer treatments, I've made some changes in my own eating plan. I do this for two reasons: to get vibrant health so I can be alert and active into my golden years and also to prevent cancer.

I actually follow the eating plan I recommend for cancer patients in chapter four. It's good for everybody! And one of the most important aspects of this diet is a mixture of flax oil and cottage cheese — an amazing discovery of the great German scientist, Johanna Budwig, Ph.D.

Since January of 2003 I've been following "the Budwig protocol" <u>every day without fail</u>. The mixture of cottage cheese and flax oil travels right to the cell membrane and repairs it. It gives the cell exactly what it needs in terms of essential fatty acids. Dr. Budwig found that cottage cheese is the ideal and most efficient carrier for flax oil. When you mix the two together, they combine into a new molecule that's uniquely capable of reforming the permeability of the cell membrane. This kills cancer cells.

Changing my eating plan and taking some supplements have changed my life and my health. Here are just a few of the changes:

- I used to get at least one or two colds every year. But I haven't had a cold in over 15 years. Why? Because my immune system is as strong as iron!
- I used to get the flu every year. But I haven't had the flu for over 15 years. Nor have I had any flu shots during that time. (Flu shots and other vaccinations contain harmful and toxic substances.)
- I've lost weight and kept it off for 15 years. My weight is ideal for my height. Yet I'm not "on a diet," and I don't feel deprived or hungry. The secret is a healthy eating plan you can live with long term, as I describe in chapter four.
- I used to have trouble sleeping, but now I sleep like a baby.
- I used to run out of steam in the afternoon, but now my energy level is high throughout the day.
- I'm mentally sharp. In fact, I play bridge on the Internet with people all over the world.
- I regularly sing in a quartet.
- I'm physically active, and I no longer have aches and pains.

That's not bad for a guy who's 80 years old, wouldn't you agree?

Don't be surprised if you experience major health benefits when you follow the eating plan and the regimen of supplements I mention in chapters four and five. It's not just a matter of preventing, avoiding, or healing cancer. It's a matter of enjoying vibrant health!

"But don't American cancer treatments *sometimes* work?"

You may be wondering why American doctors would recommend surgery, radiation, and chemo for cancer if they didn't work at least some of the time.

It's true that the harsh American cancer treatments work about two percent of the time in advanced cases of cancer. In other words, if you take 100 cancer patients at stage four (the worst stage) and if they all submit to surgery, radiation, and chemo, only two of the 100 will be alive after five years. Ninety-eight will be dead.

That means the harsh treatments that Americans take for granted have a 98 percent failure rate for late-stage cancer. But still,

these treatments have a two percent *success* rate. The explanation is the "placebo effect".

As you may know, a placebo is a fake medicine that the patient believes is real. The patient is absolutely convinced that the placebo will work — even though there's no real medicine in it.

And studies have proven the power of the placebo effect. It's real. Placebos assist the body in healing because they affect the patient's state of mind.

Many people also believe effective medicine is supposed to be unpleasant: the more unpleasant, the more effective. Because of this belief, some cancer patients may truly believe the harsh cancer treatments will work. And this belief helps a few of them survive.

That's why America's leading alternative doctor, Dr. Julian Whitaker, M.D., calls chemotherapy a "dangerous placebo". The typical placebo is harmless; it's like a "blank" that contains nothing to either harm or help the patient physically. But chemotherapy is poison. It can really hurt the cancer patient — especially when given in high doses, as doctors typically do in America. It can and does kill.

And the reason just about every cancer doctor in America recommends expensive chemotherapy drugs — some costing $10,000 a month or more! — is because they make a lot of money prescribing these drugs.

You don't have to take my word for that. An article in the *Journal of the American Medical Association* reported that the average oncologist makes $253,000 per year. Incredible as it sounds, the article says that 75 percent of those earnings — about $190,000 — come from chemotherapy drug profits! If you subtract those drug profits, the oncologist would make little more than $60,000 per year.

How to become smarter than your oncologist

The cancer patient in America today faces several choices. One choice is to do what my late wife and I did. We trusted the cancer doctors and followed their treatment plan to the letter. We put my wife's fate in the doctors' hands. They called all the shots, and we didn't question any of their decisions or recommendations.

In hindsight, I can see that was the worst mistake of our lives.

Another choice is to become smarter than the oncologist and take your health into your own hands. You might wonder how it's possible to become smarter than an oncologist — someone who spent years studying medicine and specializing in cancer.

Believe it or not, if you spend 10 or 20 hours doing research on the Internet and reading my book, you'll know more *useful* information about cancer than your oncologist. That's because the oncologist has spent all of those years studying drugs. And drugs aren't the answer. Rather, drugs are part of the problem.

A cancer patient who has decided to become smarter than the oncologist also faces another decision: whether or not to use the services of a clinic that uses alternative treatments. This is an individual decision, and there's no right or wrong answer. I've coached many clients who've defeated their cancer without the help of a clinic. I've also coached many who've gone to an alternative clinic to get rid of their cancer.

If you want to go to an alternative clinic to get rid of your cancer and if you have the money to pay for it, by all means do so. If you can't afford an alternative clinic, you can get rid of your cancer by following my seven-point plan, which I describe later in this Special Report.

Throughout this Special Report I'll mention the names of some clinics and health practitioners who've helped my clients. Some use natural remedies only, while others use a combination of standard treatments and natural remedies.

Where to get more information you can use right away

My intention in writing this Special Report is to give you practical information you can use *right now* to reverse your cancer. This Special Report lays out a plan that's simple and effective, and it gives you options so you can make an informed choice.

For lots of other good information and advice that's FREE, I invite you to log onto my website: www.beating-cancer-gently.com. If you'd like information about a wide variety of alternative cancer remedies, you may want to read my best-selling book *Cancer-Free: Your Guide to Gentle, Non-toxic Healing*. You can order it as an e-book or as a paperback book by clicking this link: www.naturalcancerremedies.com/fourthedition/

Chapter Two

The little-known link between root canals and cancer

Boston management consultant Will R. didn't have to go to the doctor to know he had cancer. He knew he had cancer when he started bleeding through his rectum in 2002. He was in his late 50s when this happened.

A medical examination confirmed Will's strong suspicion: it was colorectal cancer. Doctors found a two-centimeter tumor.

But cancer was just one of Will's many health problems. He also suffered from:

- Frequent, splitting headaches
- Severe sleep apnea and heavy snoring, causing him to wake up in the middle of the night as if he were about to choke
- Intense pain in the roof of his mouth
- Fatigue
- Fungus on his feet, back, and abdomen
- Dimming eyesight
- Night sweats so bad the sheets were soaking wet
- Twitching when he dozed off or fell asleep

Will didn't want to go under the knife. He wanted to try alternative therapies to get rid of his cancer. But the surgeon scared him onto the operating table by telling him, "You'll die without surgery." He had the operation in October of 2002.

Of course, doctors practically insisted that Will take radiation and chemotherapy. But he refused because he believed alternative treatments would be more effective.

Will became better educated about cancer than his oncologist. He read more than a dozen books about cancer, and two key facts popped out at him:

1) To beat cancer, you have to make your body as healthy as possible by natural methods. To reach this state of health, it's necessary to get rid of other diseases and infections in your body.

2) You can't be healthy if you have dead teeth such as root canal teeth, infected teeth, or infected cavitations in the jaw.

Root canals are safe, right? Wrong!

In 2003 a biological dentist examined Will and found several severe problems. (Biological dentists are mavericks who regard root canals, mercury and fluoride as harmful.) Will's two root canals were infected with staph and strep. The dentist confirmed these infections by laboratory analysis.

But Will's jaw had other problems, too. During his 20s when his wisdom teeth were extracted, the dentist failed to remove all of the connective tissues. As a result, the sockets didn't heal properly but became infected with staph and strep. This kind of dental problem following a crude extraction of a tooth is called a cavitation.

Because of his cavitations, Will had serious necrosis of the jaw — in other words, gangrene!

And the trouble with these toxic pockets in his jaw is that the staph and strep were spreading throughout Will's body, causing all kinds of health ailments. Will's root canals and the improper extraction of his wisdom teeth had caused his colorectal cancer.

Not only did the biological dentist fix Will's jaw, but he also replaced Will's mercury fillings with biologically compatible fillings.

As you know, mercury is one of the most toxic substances known to man: a teaspoon of mercury can poison a whole lake. Yet the dental establishment *still* claims that mercury is a wonderful substance for filling cavities.

The American Dental Association (ADA) has been peddling the "mercury is safe" message to the public for decades, and it's too stubborn to admit it was wrong. It's in denial about mercury, just as it's in denial about root canals.

After the biological dentist fixed Will's teeth, his health made a 180-degree turnaround:

- His cancer went into remission.
- His frequent headaches went away.
- His intense pain in the roof of his mouth went away.
- His fatigue went away.
- His fungus went away.
- His heavy night sweats stopped.
- His nighttime twitching stopped.
- His sleep apnea went away.
- His heavy snoring stopped.
- He stopped waking up in a panic with a choking feeling.
- His eyesight improved.

Will's oncologist was so impressed with his recovery from cancer that he told him, "You're the longest-living person I have who hasn't done conventional therapy. Your life expectancy was six months. There's no one like you that we know about!"

The main thing that helped Will, without a doubt, was getting his root canal teeth removed, getting his infected cavitations cleaned out, and having his mercury fillings replaced with a biologically compatible material.

"But are *all* root canals bad?"

You might be wondering whether root canals are *always* bad. Yes, they are. They're not safe. If someone with a root canal seems to be in good health, you can be sure that the person's immune system is strong enough to fight off the toxicity from the root canal. But when that same person encounters severe stress, such as a job loss, divorce, or the death of a loved one, the immune system may become weak. When the body can no longer fight off the toxicity from a root canal, a disease such as cancer can break out.

As for wisdom tooth extractions, the dentist often fails to remove all of the connective tissue from the socket. This is what leads to cavitations. Cavitations and root canals cause necrosis of the jaw: gangrene. And these dental problems contribute to perhaps half of the cancer cases in America.

"Fish story" explains what causes cancer

Here's a "fish story" that explains the cancer disaster in America.

Half the catfish in the Anacostia River in Washington, D.C., have cancerous tumors in their livers. The Anacostia River is little more than a toxic waste dump. Located within the city limits, this small, slow-moving river catches all of the nasty runoff from the city. It's actually a wonder that any fish live in it at all.

The catfish in the Anacostia River eliminate toxins and poisons through their livers. Normally, this wouldn't be a problem, but there's so much pollution that the catfish are taking in poisons faster than their livers can process and eliminate them. So how would you "cure" an Anacostia River catfish of

its liver tumors? With surgery? With toxic chemotherapy? With a liver transplant? Even if these treatments were feasible, what good would they do if we just put the "cured" catfish back into the filthy river?

It's a fact that people with cancer — like the Anacostia River catfish — have too much toxicity in their bodies. It's necessary to avoid taking in more toxins and to get rid of the toxicity that's already inside.

Using a healthy, organic eating plan helps the body get rid of many poisons. But a healthy diet won't do anything to fix an infected jawbone or a toxic root canal tooth.

Visualize a wisdom tooth being extracted. If the dentist or oral surgeon fails to remove the connecting ligament or leaves in too much bone, the gum and jaw won't heal properly. With the tooth missing, anaerobic bacteria can start growing in the hole, and this becomes even more toxic than botulism. This toxicity can get into the bloodstream and cause breast cancer, prostate cancer, and other types of cancer.

In fact, when a woman has cancer in one breast, you'll often find that the culprit is a root canal *on the same side as the cancerous breast*!

There can no longer be any doubt about the connection between root canals and cancer. I've had experience with over 3,500 cancer patients. When these cancer patients get their mouths cleaned up, they get well — even if they've tried everything else.

Pioneer dentist proved root canal toxicity in 1920s

Early in the 1900s, Dr. Weston Price, a pioneer dentist, discovered and proved that root canals are highly toxic. Dr. Price is considered one of the greatest dentists of all time. He was the head of the research arm of the precursor to the ADA.

Working with 60 other prominent dentists, Dr. Price tried to find a way to do a root canal *safely*. They worked with hundreds of patients, and tried everything under the sun. And Dr. Price concluded that there's no way to do it.

Dr. Price found that the toxicity of root canal teeth caused a wide variety of health problems, including rheumatoid arthritis, MS, cancer, glaucoma, diabetes, and so on. And he proved it with a rabbit experiment. This experiment should be famous, but the medical and dental establishment wants to drop it down the memory hole.

Here's how the experiment worked: When Dr. Price took a root canal tooth out of a diseased patient's mouth and implanted it under the skin of a rabbit, the rabbit would quickly develop the same disease.

If the patient had glaucoma, the rabbit got glaucoma. If the patient had arthritis, the rabbit got arthritis. If the patient had cancer, the rabbit got cancer. And so on. This happened hundreds of times.

Dr. Price recommended that dentists immediately stop doing root canals.

But root canals are a good income-producer for dentists. Modern dentists in America do about 40 million root canals a year. No wonder half of all American men and a third of women can expect to eventually get cancer. Each root canal silently seeps poison into the system, often resulting in health problems.

How to tell if you have a hidden jaw infection, and where to get help

How do you know if you have an undetected infection in your jawbone from a root canal or cavitation? A biological dentist can help you find out.

One way to find a biological dentist is through the International Academy of

Biological Dentistry and Medicine. Just log onto this website: www.IABDM.org and click the link for "Find a Biological Health Professional".

Another way to find a biological dentist is through the directory put together by a biological dentist, Dr. Hal Huggins, and Dr. Thomas Levy, a cardiologist who is an expert in dental toxicity. You can access this directory by calling Dr. Huggins' office at 866-948-4638 (Mountain Time). WARNING: If you call this number, don't mention anything about your cancer unless you want to get a sales pitch for Dr. Huggins' $6,000 "Blood Cleansing" program, which I consider unnecessary. Just say you want a referral to a biological dentist near you.

Incidentally, Dr. Huggins and Dr. Levy did a six-year study together from 1994 to 2000. They removed over 5,000 root canal filled teeth and tested every one of them in a lab. Dr. Levy told me that every one of them had toxins coming out of them that were "more toxic than botulism."

Chapter Three
A hidden cause of many cancers: emotional shock or stress

Teresa M., a 49-year-old woman from Toronto, has been married to the same man since she was 21. She and her husband have three children, and she works as an administrator.

She thought she was in good health, but in 2007 she experienced unusually heavy bleeding. She thought it would get better, but it didn't.

The bleeding became so bad she was rushed to the hospital, where she collapsed. She was bleeding to death. A doctor later told her, "You came within an hour of your death." The diagnosis was uterine fibroids. Doctors recommended surgery and a partial hysterectomy.

Teresa asked the doctors, "Could this be cancer?" They replied, "No."

She did have the surgery. And that's when doctors found that Teresa had endometrial cancer. Following surgery, the doctors recommended radiation, and she submitted to it out of fear.

In Teresa's medical chart, one of her doctors wrote, "Her decimation will be rapid." Her doctors basically gave up on her.

But Teresa didn't give up on herself. She began to realize that the radiation "therapy" was doing her no good whatsoever. She now says that radiation is just a theatrical exercise in which doctors put on a show that they're trying to do something for the cancer patient.

When the doctors tried to push chemotherapy on her, she said, "No! Absolutely not!"

Teresa read my best-selling book *Cancer-Free: Your Guide to Gentle, Non-toxic Healing*, and it changed her life. Here's what she tells other cancer patients:

"When you read Bill Henderson's book, your therapy will pick *you*. It will jump out at you. It's a mistake to think that there's nothing you can do about your cancer. It's also a mistake to think the doctor knows everything about you and your cancer. He doesn't! He doesn't know why it's there or what to do. That's *your* job. The good news is that you can fix it."

"Cancer will only kill you if you let it"

Teresa offers additional insights about cancer:

"It's a big mistake to try to fight your cancer. It's here to tell you something, not to kill you. It'll only kill you if you let it. Cancer is telling you that something isn't working in your life, and you have to change that. Some people would rather die than change. I'm not the same person I was several years ago.

"I feel more happiness than ever in my life. For me, cancer was a good thing because to cure myself I had to learn some lessons. And that was a blessing. I was terminal. The doctors offered no hope. My chances were nearly zero."

Teresa hopes that more cancer patients will take their lives into their own hands instead of letting the doctors do everything. She has found that taking responsibility for her own health empowered her and helped her heal.

It didn't take long for Teresa to discover that the root of her cancer was an emotional issue. She told me, "My disease was *all* emotional. There were conflicts with my adult children still living at home. Because of these conflicts I was checking out of my life and fading away. But I recognized what was happening to me and fixed it."

Teresa told me that the books she read about the mind-body connection were the most powerful help in her healing process. She specifically recommends *The Emotion Code* by Dr. Bradley B. Nelson.

Teresa is living proof that you don't need to spend years getting psychoanalyzed on a psychiatrist's couch for $100 to $200 an hour to heal yourself of emotional issues.

Cancer often makes its appearance when someone is under stress because of an emotional shock like divorce, the death of a loved one, or losing a job. But the right book can teach you how to reduce and manage the stress so that healing can begin.

Negative thinking can sabotage any treatment program and therefore must be avoided. Indeed, no doctor or treatment program can help cancer patients who believe the cancer is going to kill them. Fortunately, recent discoveries in mind-body medicine can help change this thinking.

The ultimate mind-body medicine kit

Make no mistake. Mind-body medicine is powerful. And I'm not just talking about "the power of positive thinking". Mind-body medicine is much deeper than superficial psychology. And it's real. Your mind really can help rally the healing forces within your body to defeat cancer!

The pioneer of mind-body medicine is the great physician O. Carl Simonton, M.D. Dr. Simonton's groundbreaking book *Getting Well Again* has saved many lives by educating patients about the self-awareness techniques he discovered. I can't recommend Dr. Simonton highly enough.

You can get Dr. Simonton's life-saving "Patient Package" from his website: www.simontoncenter.com. It includes two of Dr. Simonton's books and four CDs, and this information could certainly save your life or the life of a loved one.

The California man who said NO to prostate surgery

Another cancer patient with a remarkable story of recovery from cancer is Tom K., a 69-year-old man who lives in Universal City, California. I've been coaching Tom for the last couple of years, and he's eager to share his story with others.

In 2001 Tom was diagnosed with prostate cancer. A surgeon recommended surgical removal of the prostate. Tom initially agreed, and the surgery was scheduled for the following Friday.

On the Monday before the surgery, a friend urged Tom to explore some alternatives before submitting to the surgery. Tom quickly realized that there were some other options to consider and that there was no urgent need to get on the operating table.

When Tom cancelled the surgery, the surgeon was shocked. He tried to talk Tom back into it, but Tom stood firm.

Why adult diapers outsell baby diapers in America

Prostate surgery is delicate and risky. It's all too easy for the surgeon to slice nerves that control sexual and bladder functions, making the patient impotent or incontinent or both. Prostate surgery may be one reason why adult diapers now outsell baby diapers in America!

In Tom's search for an alternative, he came across Larry Clapp's protocol for prostate cancer, which in many ways is similar to what I recommend.

Larry's prostate cancer story is similar to Tom's. When Larry was diagnosed with prostate cancer in 1990, his urologist applied heavy pressure to rush him onto the operating table for surgical removal of his prostate. Larry refused. His doctor became angry and told him he would be dead within months without "proper treatment". But Larry proved his doctor wrong.

And so did Tom.

Tom later discovered my best-selling book *Cancer-Free: Your Guide to Gentle, Non-toxic Healing*, and he decided to hire me as his cancer coach. We often exchange e-mails and phone calls.

Tom believes one cause of his cancer was tension and stress. He was having a lot of trouble with a neighbor who became a complete "jerk". Tom had already endured a lot of stress, and he figures his neighborhood "jerk" was the straw that broke the camel's back.

To heal himself of stress, Tom used the Emotional Freedom Technique (EFT). He says EFT defused his irrational emotional experiences, enabling him to live freely and to feel comfortable in his own skin. He also hired a hypno-therapist in Palm Springs, and he found that therapy helpful.

In addition to stress management, Tom found out that he needed to have some root canals removed. He found a biological dentist in the Los Angeles area, Harold E. Ravins, D.D.S., and hired him to do the necessary work. Dr. Ravins's address is 12381 Wilshire Blvd # 103, Los Angeles, CA 90025. His office phone number is 310-207-4617.

But Tom needed more than just the removal of his root canals. Dr. Ravins also removed his mercury fillings (the so-called "silver amalgam" fillings) and replaced them with biologically compatible fillings.

Tom has found that knowledge is power. He says that just knowing about the alternatives to chemo and surgery was the most important thing that helped him. He now understands the nature of cancer, which is only a symptom that the body isn't working right.

Tom is convinced that fixing his root canals helped strengthen his immune system. And he further strengthened it by improving his nutrition. He follows my recommendations for supplements as described in chapter five of this Special Report. And he also follows the eating plan I recommend in chapter four, including Dr. Budwig's flax oil/cottage cheese mixture.

When Tom's M.D. examined him, he could only agree that Tom was on the right path. He told him, "Keep on doing what you're doing."

Tom offers some advice for cancer patients: "Keep an open mind. You have good options. And hire a cancer coach."

I certainly have enjoyed coaching Tom. The last time I spoke to him, he said, "My health is incredible. My spirit is good."

Let me close this chapter by pointing out that the simplest and cheapest way to fix emotional issues is to read and apply the ideas in *The Emotion Code* by Dr. Bradley B. Nelson. This book costs less than $20, and you don't need to work with a professional to apply the ideas. You can fix emotional issues yourself.

The Emotional Freedom Technique (EFT), by contrast, usually requires a professional. And that's more expensive. That's why I recommend you try *The Emotion Code* first. If that doesn't work, you could try EFT. You can learn more about it at www.emofree.com.

Chapter Four
Change your eating plan and *save your life!*

Too many Americans are digging their own graves with their teeth. That's because the typical American diet today is practically guaranteed to cause diseases including cancer. The obvious culprits are such things as refined sugar, high fructose corn syrup, hormone-laden meats, pesticide-tainted fruits and vegetables, and processed foods with an ever-expanding list of artificial preservatives and additives.

It shouldn't be surprising that eating these foods on a daily basis creates a toxic load within the body. Several organs of the human body are designed to help the body get rid of toxins. These cleansing organs include the liver, the kidneys, the lungs, the skin, and the colon. But the human body runs into trouble when it takes in poisons faster than it can get rid of them.

To fix that imbalance and get rid of the toxic buildup, the cancer patient in America today must do two things: reduce as much as possible the intake of toxins and get rid of the toxins that have built up over the years.

And there's a surprisingly simple way to accomplish that. Change your eating plan.

Practically all of my clients have done that, and the results are astonishing. Consider what happened to one of my clients, Sandra G. of Little Rock.

Sandra had stage-four breast cancer, which many doctors consider terminal. But Sandra rejected the doctor's death sentence and got busy healing herself.

Today she's in vibrant health without a trace of cancer. She says the secret of her success is her new eating plan, which put the right things into her body and helped get rid of the bad stuff that had built up.

Sandra says, "The new eating plan will detoxify you. This is almost embarrassing to say, but when I started on the new eating plan, it was almost like the toxins were coming out of my pores. I could kind of smell myself."

Sandra's battle with breast cancer began in 1994 when she was first diagnosed with it. She didn't know about any alternatives at the time, so she went along with the standard treatments such as chemo.

But the cancer came back. Sandra started looking for alternatives so she wouldn't have to go through the agony of chemotherapy again. She came across my book, changed her eating plan, and got rid of her cancer.

Sandra was cancer-free for two years, and then she let down her guard and went back to her old eating habits. She learned the hard way what a mistake that was.

In April of 2008, her doctor told her, "You have two months to live." And when the doctor saw her again in September, he repeated, "You have two months to live." Apparently he forgot that that's what he had told her five months earlier. Like a broken record, he just repeated his prediction, "You have two months to live."

Too many doctors are exactly like that. They put on their white coats and, acting like miniature gods, pronounce death sentences over their cancer patients. Sadly, when the patient takes the doctor-oracle seriously, it usually comes true.

But Sandra did have one foot in the grave: she knew death was staring her in the face. And she would have died if she hadn't made some changes. So she made a commitment right then and there to get back on the healthy eating plan and to *stay on it for life*!

When she returned for a follow-up visit to her doctor — the same one who kept telling her "you have two months to live" — even *he* was stunned that all traces of her cancer were gone! He couldn't deny it. And Sandra was ecstatic. She's confident the cancer will never return as long as she sticks to the eating plan.

Reflecting on her recovery, Sandra says, "Life is good. God is wonderful. My e-mail box is full, and my phone has been busy with people calling to ask what I did. It's a good feeling."

My six recommendations for cancer patients are the cornerstone of her eating plan:

- No sugar
- No flour
- No processed foods: if it's not in the form God made it, you don't eat it!
- No meat or fish. After you've overcome cancer, you can have *some* organic meat and fish, but red meat should be avoided.
- No dairy except for the cottage cheese you mix with flax oil
- Lots of organic fruits and vegetables — especially vegetables. *Raw* vegetables are highly recommended.

Finding organic fruits and vegetables can be difficult, but it's worth the effort.

As an integral part of this eating plan, Sandra practically swears by the Budwig protocol — the mixture of flax oil and cottage cheese. In chapter one, I mentioned Johanna Budwig, Ph. D., and her discovery that eating a mixture of cottage cheese and flax oil can heal cancer.

You may be thinking: "But isn't cottage cheese a dairy product, and don't you claim that cancer patients should avoid dairy?" Yes, cottage cheese *is* a dairy product, but when you thoroughly mix it with flax oil as I recommend, it loses all of its dairy properties. I've repeatedly found that people who suffer from dairy intolerance have absolutely no problem eating the cottage cheese/flaxseed oil mixture.

The best flax oil on the market is Barlean's, which you can get at Whole Foods or order directly from the company (www.barleans.com). Once you've got it, mix it with cottage cheese as follows:

For a therapeutic dose, take one-third of a cup of flax oil and two thirds of a cup of cottage cheese and mix it well together in a bowl and let the mixture sit for five to eight minutes. Then put the mixture in a blender and add berries and walnuts and almonds. Add some stevia as a sweetener, if you like. Add some water, if necessary. Mix it in a blender on the "Liquefy" setting. Do this every morning.

Once you've gotten rid of your cancer, you should keep on doing the Budwig protocol, but you can scale back to a maintenance dose: use about half the amount of flax oil and cottage cheese you were using for the therapeutic dose.

Sandra says she took the therapeutic dose until she had been cancer-free for six months, and then she went to the maintenance dose, which she'll stay on for life. That's smart. That's the way to keep cancer from ever coming back.

For more information about Dr. Budwig's life-saving formula, Sandra *strongly* recommends the website www.budwig-videos.com. She credits this website with

helping to save her life. And it's not just about the Budwig mixture of flax oil and cottage cheese. It contains lots of great advice for a healthy eating plan you can live with for the rest of your life.

Sandra doesn't just stop at taking the flax oil. She also incorporates several other health practices into her new, cancer-free lifestyle, including:

- Laetrile (amygdalin), which is refined from apricot seeds. Sandra obtains a Laetrile product called "Amygdalina" from a Mexican pharmacy. She orders it online from www.cytopharmaonline.com and she believes it has helped her. The pharmacy's e-mail address is info@cytopharmaonline.com. Its toll-free phone number is 1-888-271-4184.

- Essiac tea. This tea, popularized by the Canadian nurse Renee Caisse in the 1920s, is a traditional American Indian remedy for cancer. (Essiac is "Caisse" spelled backwards.) This tea consists of four herbs: burdock root, slippery elm bark, sheep sorrel, and Indian or Turkish rhubarb root. Sandra buys the fresh herbs and makes her own tea. Many health food stores sell Essiac tea already made.

- Coffee enemas. The concept of coffee enemas might sound strange to you, but medical studies have proven that coffee enemas help flush and detoxify the liver. Coffee enemas can assist a healthy diet in detoxification.

- The regimen of supplements I recommend. (See chapter five for a complete description of these supplements.)

Sandra emphasizes that cancer patients must commit to permanent lifestyle changes or else cancer will come back with a vengeance. She had to learn that lesson the hard way, and she came close to dying as a result. She plans to be on the Budwig protocol for life, and she expects to live into her golden years in good health.

Businesswoman from San Diego said NO to chemotherapy

Lynda C. is a business coach from San Diego, California. She was 42 when she noticed a lump on her breast. "It was huge — like the end of a thumb," says Linda. That happened in July of 2006.

At first, her doctor denied that it was cancer. He told her, "Don't worry about it." But several weeks later the lump became painful. A surgeon removed the lump, which was about the size of a grape. A couple days after the surgery, the surgeon gave Lynda the shocking news that "there was cancer in that lump."

So the surgeon scheduled more surgery. In the second surgery he took out a cue-ball size amount of breast tissue. Lynda says, "The surgery left me deformed."

Following up on the surgery, Lynda's oncologist insisted on aggressive chemotherapy. Like a used car salesman, he pushed it. And he wouldn't take no for an answer. Lynda asked the oncologist, "What can I do to strengthen my immune system?" The oncologist replied, "Nothing. It would hurt the chemo. We have to do aggressive chemotherapy!"

Lynda replied, "Thank you very much. I won't need your services."

This rejection shocked the chemotherapy oncologist, who continued harassing Lynda for two more months, trying to get her to submit to his chemo. Finally he gave up.

When Lynda went to the radiation oncologist, he told her, "I'd like to help you, but you're not a candidate for radiation. We don't know what to radiate in your case." So Lynda avoided both chemotherapy and radiation.

Instead, she opted for reconstructive breast surgery, which she found empowering.

Lynda resisted reading my book *Cancer-Free: Your Guide to Gentle, Non-toxic Healing* because she comes from a science background, and she's skeptical. But once she started reading it, she devoured it. And she read other books, too, such as *Root Canal Cover-up* and a book about Laetrile. She totally committed herself to my seven-point program, as described in chapter five of this Special Report. Blood tests indicated Lynda was cancer-free. And so she assumed she was out of danger and went back to some of her earlier habits.

Lynda's mother died about a month later — in July of 2008 — and by August Lynda developed a pain in her right shoulder. It turned out to be cancer, and this time her oncologist recommended radiation. Although Lynda was scared, she decided to hold off on radiation treatments. She told the oncologist, "Give me eight weeks" and she made an appointment for a follow-up visit eight weeks later.

When Lynda got back in touch with me to discuss what to do about the return of her cancer, I told her she needed to get back on my seven-point program — especially the Budwig protocol of flax oil and cottage cheese! She immediately got back on the straight and narrow.

The amazing fruit seeds that kill cancer *and* pain

To get rid of her pain and control her cancer, Lynda also decided to add apricot seeds for the amygdalin — the main ingredient in Laetrile. You can buy apricot seeds by the bag over the Internet from websites such as www.apricotpower.com or www.cancerchoices.com.

Many people know that Laetrile is a cancer remedy. But few people know about its wonderful pain-killing effects.

Lynda eats about 50 apricot seeds a day, but she says it's a big mistake to eat them all at once. "Don't eat more than about seven at a time," she cautions, "or else you may feel a palpitation and your heart might race or beat hard."

Lynda once made the mistake of eating 50 apricot seeds all at once. She put the 50 seeds in a blender and mixed them with her flax oil/cottage cheese shake. But she got more than she bargained for, including a pounding in her ears, dizziness, the shakes, and inability to focus. "It was ugly," Lynda says. So she decided to scale back her apricot seed intake to seven at a time.

Now Lynda eats seven apricot seeds at a time without any problem, and she does this seven times a day. She practically swears by it as a natural painkiller. She has had no shoulder pain since eating the apricot seeds.

My seven-point program and the apricot seeds must be working for Lynda, because when she went in for her follow-up visit, her oncologist found no trace of cancer. Consequently, he recommended no radiation! Instead, he told her, "Keep doing what you're doing!" And then he stopped to ask, "What *are* you doing?" She replied, "Apricot seeds." He answered, "I've heard good things about those."

If only all doctors were as curious and as open-minded as Lynda's oncologist.

Cajun plantation owner recalls, "I had one foot in the grave"

The doctors offered no hope to seventh-generation plantation owner Richard L., a Cajun from Brusly, Louisiana, across the Mississippi River from Baton Rouge. Sixty-

one-year-old Richard told me, "I had one foot in the grave, and the other on a banana peel."

He wasn't joking.

Richard suffered from a brain tumor just behind his eye. His medical troubles actually began back in 1991 when he had water in his eye and a detached retina. His doctor recommended surgery and described it as a "piece of cake". Richard replied, "Do it." After surgery, Richard was blinded in his right eye.

In 1998 Richard went back to his doctor because of pain in that eye. The diagnosis was cancer. Richard's doctors removed his eye and gave him seven weeks of radiation, which caused unbearable headaches for two and three weeks at a time.

He said the headaches were "hell". Richard had no more trouble until early 2006 when he had trouble keeping his balance. The cancer had returned. It was brain cancer behind his eye. His doctors operated to remove the cancer, and they also removed part of Richard's brain covering, the "dura mater".

In February 2006, Richard's doctors gave him the bleak prediction that he had two to six months to live. Richard wasn't happy with that prognosis, so he sought a second opinion. But the grim prognosis was the same.

So Richard checked out of the hospital and checked into a hospice. The doctors put him on morphine, and he prepared for death.

Normally, when someone checks into a hospice, it's the end of the line. They don't "check out" except to go to the cemetery.

Richard's turnaround: from hospice to health

But when I interviewed Richard three years later, he was happy to be back home on his plantation. Richard told me, "Bill, if it weren't for you, I wouldn't have made it. I wouldn't be alive today."

I'll never forget the day Richard called me from his hospice. He was lying down on his couch, and he asked what I would recommend. Without hesitation, I recommended the simple seven-point program I describe in chapter five of this special report. Richard ordered the supplements and started with the program.

Richard's steady improvement astounded the hospice personnel and the doctors, who almost never see patients get up and walk out of the hospice.

Richard told me, "You have to stick to the healthy eating plan 100 percent or you're wasting your time. You can't have any red meat — NONE! I'll have some chicken, turkey, fish, and some rabbit once in a while."

At five feet 10.5 inches, Richard had been down to a shocking 119 pounds. Because of the healthy eating plan, he gained 15 pounds.

And Richard told me he's helped quite a few other people get rid of cancer. Lots of people want to know how he did it.

He told me, "Some people are hard to convince. I've put quite a few people on flax oil and cottage cheese. Some quit, and some are still doing it. They have to want to do it. If they don't want to do it, there's no hope for them. I know people who've refused to eat flax oil and cottage cheese. And guess what: they're dead!"

From the brink of the grave to survival!

In the year 2000, Marilou P., a teacher from Montreal, noticed an anomaly in her breast. Her doctor said it was nothing. But it grew. A year later another doctor told her it was metastasized breast cancer. She had a complete mastectomy that included removal of the lymph nodes.

Marilou's doctor gave her six months to live

in 2001. The cancer even spread to her lungs, making the outlook even more bleak. She could hardly breathe or walk. After taking just five steps, she was completely out of breath. Her husband Franco said she looked about 80 years old, even though she was only 35.

Just when it seemed there was no hope at all, Franco came across my book *Cancer-Free*. Considering that Franco's wife was under a death sentence, he figured she had nothing to lose by trying the protocol I recommend. So he started giving his wife cottage cheese mixed with flax oil every day.

The results were astounding. Within one month the lung cancer completely disappeared. Her youthful appearance returned, and she was able to walk without any problem whatsoever. Franco says, "It's unbelievable how fast the lung cancer left."

When Marilou survived five years after her doctor's death sentence, she knew she was cancer free. Her survival story is an encouragement to cancer survivors everywhere.

Ten-year breast cancer survivor was told: "You'll be dead in a year"

Doctors didn't give Wiltrude much hope when they diagnosed her with cancer in the year 2000. Wiltrude, a psychologist from Germany, never thought cancer would happen to her. But it did. And it came as a big shock.

One doctor told her, "You'll be dead in a year."

Wiltrude didn't have much money for expensive cancer treatments like radiation and chemo. When she told a doctor she was going to try alternative treatments, her doctor said, "You are committing suicide with what you are doing." But she was determined to find a way to beat her cancer.

Somehow Wiltrude came across my book *Cancer-Free*. It made perfect sense to her, especially the Budwig Protocol (flax oil/cottage cheese) that I recommend. She made the Budwig Protocol a part of her daily routine.

Not only has Wiltrude passed the five-year cancer survival mark, she has survived 10 years. The radiologist who tests her every year told her, "You're the only one with this kind of result." Indeed, most women who have the kind of breast cancer Wiltrude had don't survive very long.

"My wife would be dead by now if I had listened to her doctors"

Stuart and Sara S. are a married couple in their late 50s. They both grew up in Hawaii, but now they're living in Monterey County, south of San Francisco.

Back in 2001 Sara was diagnosed with breast cancer and had a lumpectomy. This health crisis inspired her husband to embark on a cancer research project similar to the one I embarked on following my first wife's death. During his research, he made discoveries similar to those I had made.

Stuart eagerly shared his research and his wife's success story with me. And I'm happy to pass on this life-saving information to you.

In 2005 doctors found cancer in Sara's lymph nodes and also in her bones. The cancer was back with a vengeance, and the prognosis was bad. Once cancer has spread to your bones, you're pretty well through, according to most cancer doctors. But Stuart says, "I apparently found a cure for my wife's metastatic bone cancer. It was natural, and it worked."

Stuart says, "Had I listened to Sara's doctors, my wife would be dead by now." Instead, his wife applied the natural cure Stuart had discovered, which kicks the

immune system into high gear. A healthy immune system nips cancer cells in the bud. But when the immune system is weak, cancer cells run loose and multiply.

It became obvious to Stuart that the way to save Sara's life was to strengthen her immune system — especially the Natural Killer (NK) cells that kill cancer cells without harming healthy cells.

Stuart was shocked to find out that chemotherapy weakens or destroys the immune system. Among other things, chemotherapy kills NK cells. And he's flabbergasted that any doctor would even suggest chemotherapy as a treatment for cancer.

The four natural products that cured Stuart's wife

There's only one way to cure cancer, according to Stuart: build up the body's immune system so it can kill the cancer. A healing method must increase the strength of the NK cells in the body and escalate their level of activity. This healing must also unmask the cancer cells, which can be quite clever at disguising themselves from the immune system.

Stuart believes that he has found such a healing process. Although he doesn't claim that it will heal *every* case of cancer, it certainly worked for his wife's cancer, which doctors had called "terminal".

Whether you want to heal cancer, build up your immune system, improve the quality of your health, or do all of these things, Stuart strongly recommends four natural products. These are the same four his wife took. She's been cancer-free for four years since she started taking them.

"Her cancer almost miraculously disappeared — even from her bones — within two months of starting the regimen," says Stuart, "and according to PET scans and other sophisticated testing, her cancer has not since returned. Sara used to get two colds a year, but she hasn't been sick with anything."

The four natural products that cured Sara are Avemar, Immune-Assist, Transfer Factor Plus, and Cell Forte. When Stuart tells people about this cure, he encourages them to look up information about each of the four products on the Internet.

The first product Stuart recommends is Avemar, which got its name from "Ave Maria" ("Hail Mary" in Latin). In America the name of the product is usually shortened to "Ave." It's available from American Biosciences (www.americanbiosciences.com; 888-884-7770). Stuart says Avemar works by unmasking the cancer cells so your NK cells can identify them as enemies and destroy them.

Stuart doesn't like the taste of Avemar, but he says Sara is used to it.

To boost your immune system, Stuart recommends Immune-Assist from Aloha Medicinals (www.alohamedicinals.com). It contains mushroom extracts and other natural substances that build up a powerful immune-system army of NK cells. And Stuart says you can increase the strength of this army of NK cells by adding another product, Transfer Factor Plus, which is also available from Aloha Medicinals.

The fourth product Sara used to heal her cancer is Cell Forte, which is available from Enzymatic Therapy (800-783-2286). You may also be able to find it at your local health food store. Cell Forte stimulates the NK cells to work like crazy. It's like putting the NK cells on steroids, although Cell Forte is a completely natural product, not a drug.

Stuart says he spends about $12.50 per day

on these products. And he points out that it's a lot less expensive than chemotherapy, which would almost certainly have killed Sara. Chemo would have damaged or destroyed her immune system, allowing the cancer cells to run loose and multiply freely.

If $12.50 per day sounds too expensive, hold on. In chapter five I describe my seven-point program, which costs only about $5.15 per day.

Stuart freely shares information about his wife's amazing cancer recovery whenever he hears that someone is struggling with cancer.

For example, Stuart has a business partner who lives in Arizona. About three years ago his business partner phoned him and mentioned that his landlord's wife had late-stage cancer and wasn't expected to live. Stuart immediately sent his partner information about how Sara healed herself of "terminal" cancer so he could pass it on to the landlord. Stuart didn't think anything more of it.

But three years later — about a month before I interviewed him — Stuart got a phone call out of the blue from his partner's landlord. The landlord told Stuart, "I just want to thank you from the bottom of my heart for helping my wife get rid of her cancer." His wife had been so sick that she wasn't even able to walk. But the landlord and his wife had just come back from a hiking expedition in Europe!

The American cancer industry is silent about the various cancer cures, such as the one that healed Stuart's wife and the landlord's wife. People are learning about these healing methods through word-of-mouth advertising and through books such as mine. You could save a life just by passing on information about how to get rid of cancer with natural, non-toxic methods.

Palm Beach cancer survivor reveals secret

Rebecca K. and her husband live in Palm Beach, Florida. But during hurricane season you're more likely to find them at their yacht club in Gloucester, Massachusetts. In fact, they're so grateful for my help as a cancer coach that they recently treated my wife and me to three nights at their Gloucester yacht club.

They're absolutely convinced that I saved Rebecca's life.

Nearly 13 years ago Rebecca started suffering heavy bleeding during her periods. She was in her late 50s at the time. The bleeding got worse, and the doctors couldn't stop it. When the doctors found uterine cancer, they recommended a hysterectomy plus taking out the fallopian tubes, the ovaries — everything.

Rebecca had this operation six years ago. And her doctors wanted to follow up the operation with radiation therapy just to make sure all the cancer cells were dead. She told them, "No, thank you." She preferred to find a natural remedy to keep cancer away.

At a health fair she came across a newsletter that mentioned my book *Cancer-Free: Your Guide to Gentle, Non-toxic Healing*. She read the book and hired me as a coach.

Rebecca did my seven-point program as described in chapter five of this Special Report. And she still sticks to it religiously.

For example, she has her flax oil and cottage cheese mixture without fail *every day*. She's committed to it. She likes to add blueberries and a banana to the mixture. She says you can add just about anything. Sometimes she adds pineapple chunks and blends them up with the flax oil and cottage cheese.

Whiskey helps heal cancer?

But she did add one thing that might raise your eyebrows — a whiskey drink! Normally I don't recommend alcohol for cancer patients because alcohol feeds cancer. But Rebecca swears by her whiskey concoction.

Rebecca starts with a pound of *raw* honey, and she emphasizes that the honey must be raw. Then she adds a jigger of whiskey plus three fresh leaves of aloe (after removing the sharp ends). And then she mixes it up in a blender. Both Rebecca and her husband drink this mixture.

When I spoke to Rebecca recently, she told me, "Bill, you gave me what's the most precious thing in the world: another day — and many more!"

I love to hear testimonials like that, and I get them all the time. That's why I say that this is the most fulfilling thing I've done in my entire life. Nothing has been anywhere near as gratifying as what I do now. Every day I get an opportunity to help somebody. And what could be better than that?

Chapter Five
What I would do if *I* had cancer:
My simple seven-point program for *any* type of cancer

In this chapter I'll tell you exactly what I'd do if *I* had cancer. Actually, I'm already doing most of the seven-point program now to keep in good health. And it's working. I've lost weight and kept it off for *years*, I'm physically active with high energy, I'm mentally alert, and my immune system is as strong as iron.

Nothing succeeds like success. And health success is what I want for you and for your loved ones.

The simple program I'm about to describe has been proven over many years to work on all types of cancer. Yes, *all* types. Here's an outline of the seven points:

1. Boost your sagging immune system — Transfer Point's Beta Glucan is best.
2. The Budwig protocol: flax oil and cottage cheese — to reform the oxygen uptake of your cells.
3. Vitamin C and l-Lysine/l-Proline with Green Tea Extract — to stop the spread of the cancer.
4. Greens and enzymes — to make your body alkaline and give you the enzymes you need.
5. A cancer-fighting diet — to detox your body and restore its balance.
6. A vitamin-mineral supplement — to cover all the needed essentials.
7. Vitamin D3 -- to give an extra boost to this essential nutrient.

That's it. It's no more complicated than that. Anybody can do it. And it's so cheap that even those who can't afford health insurance can afford my seven points. In short, this is a Rolls Royce cancer treatment program for those on a Ford budget.

Believe it or not, I know people who've gotten rid of their cancer by applying just one of the seven points in my recommended treatment program. But if you apply all seven, cancer hardly stands a chance. Do I *guarantee* it will work? Sorry. No guarantees. In any case, it's your decision, and you have to take full responsibility for it. All I can do is share what I know. But if you apply my program, I would be astounded if your health doesn't improve. And when your health gets stronger, the cancer gets weaker.

Having cancer is like a teeter-totter: cancer is on one end and your health is on the other end. When you apply my program, it's normal for your health to go up and for cancer to go down, even if your doctor has given you a death sentence.

I encourage you to discuss my program with your doctor. But before you do, you must be convinced that it will work. Otherwise your doctor will tell you it's a waste of time and talk you out of it. And if your doctor isn't at least sympathetic or tolerant, you should consider finding another doctor.

How to boost your immune system and make your cancer run and hide

No cancer either begins or thrives if your immune system is strong. So your first priority,

whether you want to prevent cancer or to heal from it, is to get your immune system in cancer-fighting shape. Supplements are essential for doing that. I'll discuss diet later, but no diet should be considered adequate to *reverse* cancer. An effective cancer treatment program requires nutritional supplementation, period.

There are several options, but to keep it simple I'll just give you my first choice. It's the one *I* use. The product is called Beta-1, 3D Glucan. It's made by Transfer Point, a company in Columbia, South Carolina. I'd say this product beats other immune-boosting products hands-down. If you have cancer, you need to take one capsule for each 50 pounds (23 kilos) of body weight. Take it all in the morning, on an empty stomach.

Here are some reasons why Beta-1, 3D Glucan is a superior product:

- Almost all immune booster products are soluble. That means that it's difficult to control where they dissolve in the body and where they will have their effect. But Beta-1, 3D Glucan is in a capsule that travels where it will do the most good — namely, it passes from the stomach to the small intestine. In the small intestine it dissolves so it can enter the lymphatic system. From there, it's carried into the bloodstream by a complex process.

- Beta-1, 3D Glucan "primes" the neutrophil immune cells to recognize cancer cells and kill them. Neutrophil cells make up half or more of your immune system cells. Beta-1, 3D Glucan plants a receptor in the outer membrane of these cells. With this receptor, they "see" cancer cells as enemies and kill them dead!

- Taking the proper dose of Beta-1, 3D Glucan (depending on your weight) once a day can double the strength of your immune system. This makes it simple. In other words, there's no need to take the product several times throughout the day. Nor do you gain anything by taking more than the recommended amount.

- Some of the competing products use beta glucan from mushrooms or from cereal grains or from both. But those products are much less effective than a product like Beta-1, 3D Glucan, which gets its beta glucan from yeast.

Let me make one thing crystal clear. Though Beta-1, 3D Glucan is a yeast-based product, there's no harm in taking it. None. Specifically, it doesn't cause yeast infections like *candida albicans*. You can take this product with peace of mind as you visualize it mobilizing your immune system to kill off any nasty enemies in your body.

Beta-1, 3D Glucan is available from this special website: www.ancient5.com

I make no commission when you order this product. I recommend it because I believe in it and use it myself every day.

If you prefer to phone, just call toll-free 855-877-8220. They're in Atlanta, Georgia (Eastern time zone). Outside the U.S., you can call (678) 653-8532. Taking a potent immune system boosting product will almost certainly *ensure* that your cancer will not recur. Without boosting your immune system, your cancer will almost certainly come back months or years after you're declared "cancer-free". And you can take a product to boost your immune system whether you use alternative therapy, conventional therapy, or a combination of alternative and conventional therapies.

In short, there's no downside. But the upside potential is tremendous.

The Budwig protocol: The amazing formula that can cure cancer!

I use the Budwig protocol every day without fail because it's just about the cheapest health insurance you can buy. What does the Budwig protocol do? Well, consider this. The Budwig protocol consists of a mixture of flax oil and cottage cheese, making a unique substance that kills cancer cells by the *billions* and makes every other cell in your body healthier — *at the same time!*

In short, when a cancer patient goes on the Budwig protocol, the cancer cells get the message that the jig is up.

You don't have to take my word for it. Here's what oncologist and former cardiologist Dan C. Roehm, M.D., said:

"This diet is far and away the most successful anti-cancer diet in the world. What Dr. Johanna Budwig has demonstrated to my initial disbelief, but lately to my complete satisfaction in my practice, is this: cancer is easily curable. The treatment is dietary, and the response is immediate. The cancer cell is weak and vulnerable."

The American cancer industry doesn't want you to know how simple, how inexpensive, and how successful cancer treatment can be.

If you need more proof, here's what Robert Willner, M.D., said: "A top European cancer research scientist, Dr. Johanna Budwig, has discovered a totally natural formula that protects against the development of cancer. Furthermore, people all over the world who have been diagnosed with incurable cancer and sent home to die have actually been cured and now lead normal, healthy lives."

I eat Dr. Budwig's formula every day for prevention and to maintain peak health.

The Budwig formula is so simple and easy to make it seems ridiculous. You simply combine two-thirds of a cup of cottage cheese (ideally low-fat, organic) with one-third of a cup of fresh, refrigerated flax oil and mix it in a blender. Or you can mix it with a hand-blender (also called an "immersion blender"). Stirring isn't good enough. To mix it properly, you have to blend it.

Once you've mixed it, you can add — if you wish — whatever kind of fruit you want: strawberries, blueberries, or whatever is your favorite. You can also add something like almonds or walnuts. I don't recommend peanuts because peanuts are often heavily laden with pesticides or fungus.

Adding fruit should make the Budwig mixture sweet enough. But if you want more sweetener, just add stevia — a natural sweetener that doesn't feed cancer cells.

You may have heard that dairy products are bad for cancer patients, and I would agree with that. But when you mix cottage cheese with flax oil, it loses its dairy properties. Dozens of people I know who are lactose-intolerant eat the Budwig protocol every day without any problems whatsoever.

It's easy to find flax oil. You can get it at Whole Foods and other health food stores — for starters. And you can also get it by mail order directly from Barleans. You can call them at 800-445-3529 (Pacific Time).

Dr. Budwig's formula is used therapeutically in Europe for prevention and treatment of many diseases, including cancer, arteriosclerosis, stroke, heart attack, irregular heartbeat, stomach ulcers, arthritis, eczema, and immune deficiency syndromes such as MS and autoimmune diseases such as lupus.

If you have cancer, please don't quibble with me about Dr. Budwig's protocol. Don't wait to tell your doctor. *Just do it!*

It's food. And because it replaces one or two meals a day, it costs little or nothing. It

can't hurt you unless the oil is rancid, which would be pretty obvious. If the oil smells or tastes awful, don't eat it. Take it back and get some fresh, refrigerated Barleans flax oil.

If you have cancer, the Budwig protocol should be a *lifetime commitment*. Let me repeat that: you should use the Budwig protocol *for life*! In other words, don't flake off from using it after you get rid of your cancer. Many of my coaching clients have found out the hard way that it was a bad idea to quit the Budwig protocol. Rather, keep on using it every day without fail. You can give it plenty of variety by throwing different berries and nuts into the mixture.

How the Budwig protocol kills cancer cells by the *billions*

You may be wondering how a simple mixture of flax oil and cottage cheese could cause cancer cells to die by the billions. It happens by a complicated process, but I'll explain it in a simplified form.

As I mentioned in chapter one, cancer cells react to oxygenation the way a vampire would react to broad daylight: they shrivel up and die. And when healthy cells get more oxygen, they produce more energy, and your health becomes more vibrant.

Basically, the Budwig protocol *blasts* the cancer cells with oxygen. And it also brings more oxygen to healthy cells.

Every cell in your body needs omega 3, an essential fatty acid, both on the cell membrane and inside the cell. But the typical American doesn't get enough omega 3. According to Dr. Budwig, one of the richest sources of omega 3 is flax oil.

Omega 3 works like a magnet on the cell membrane, attracting oxygen to the cell and also causing the oxygen to enter the cell. You may have plenty of oxygen circulating in your blood, but if your cells don't have enough omega 3, the oxygen won't get into your cells.

Cells that don't get enough oxygen can become anaerobic — in other words, they find a way to live without oxygen and instead rely on sugar. These anaerobic cells stay alive and multiply through a fermentation process. Cancer cells are anaerobic. They no longer need oxygen and, in fact, can no longer stand it!

When you take the Budwig protocol, the cancer cells get an infusion of omega 3 followed by a blast of fresh oxygen, and millions of cancer cells die on a regular schedule.

Considering that flax oil is so good for you, you might decide to take it without the cottage cheese. But that would be a big mistake! Blending cottage cheese with the flax oil is a crucial part of the protocol, according to Dr. Budwig, because this mixture is the best way to deliver omega 3 to cells throughout your body. When you blend cottage cheese with the flax oil, not only does the cottage cheese lose its dairy properties, as I mentioned before, but also the mixture becomes water-soluble. This water solubility is why the Budwig protocol delivers omega 3 to the cells so efficiently and effectively.

If you have cancer, I hope you'll make a firm commitment to take the Budwig protocol and stay on it *for life*.

The vitamin C protocol that works wonders against cancer

The next treatment I'd add to my cancer-fighting regimen is a mixture of vitamin C, l-Lysine, and l-Proline. The latter two are common amino acids. Dr. Linus Pauling and Dr. Matthias Rath discovered this combination in the mid-1980s. They found that this combination inhibits the process of metastasis of cancer cells — in other words, the spread of

cancer from the original site to other organs. They also discovered that adding Green Tea Extract enhances the beneficial effect.

I recommend this treatment because it's gentle, non-toxic, and readily available. As an added bonus, it's inexpensive. The product I recommend is called Heart Plus. You can get it dirt-cheap from the same place I get it: Our Health Coop. This is my favorite source for inexpensive natural products. They charge wholesale plus five percent. Where can you get nutritional products cheaper than that?

Believe it or not, the Our Health Coop price for Heart Plus is $9.45. Is that for one day? No. It's for 180 tablets — about enough for a 30-day supply! I also recommend that you take Heart Plus with Green Tea Extract, which you can also get from Our Health Coop. A month's supply of Green Tea Extract also costs about $10.

The website for Our Health Coop is www.MakingHealthAffordable.com.

If I had cancer, I'd take six of the Heart Plus throughout the day — two capsules at a time — and three capsules of Green Tea Extract — one at a time — along with the Heart Plus.

Greens and enzymes change your body chemistry!

For cancer patients I believe greens and enzymes are essential. And one green/enzyme product I recommend without reservation is "Barley Power" from a company called Green Supreme, Inc. It comes in a 200- or 400-tablet bottle and you can get it by calling (800) 358-0777. Their local number in Pennsylvania is (724) 946-9057. You can use the local number from outside the U.S. or go to their website www.GreenSupreme.net.

One of the most beneficial things Barley Power does is to alkalize your body. Bear in mind that an acidic body is a welcoming environment for cancer and other diseases. You definitely want to alkalize your body.

And there's a simple way to determine your pH level. The same company that sells Barley Power also sells inexpensive rolls of pH test strips. An 8-foot roll costs about $10.

Here's how to use the pH test strip. Every morning when you wake up (before you eat or drink anything) you put a two-inch strip under your tongue for a couple of seconds, and it'll show where you are on the alkaline to acidic scale. The ideal is about 6.4 or higher.

If you're eating a typical American diet, your pH is probably around 5.5 or less. That's extremely acidic. The Barley Power tablets can move this number to the alkaline range in about two to three weeks.

A simple cancer-fighting eating plan

Before I describe my simple cancer-fighting eating plan, let me start out by making certain assumptions:

- You don't smoke or chew tobacco
- You don't drink sodas (either sugared sodas or so-called "diet" sodas)
- You aren't taking recreational drugs
- You aren't drinking any alcohol
- You aren't drinking anything with caffeine beyond a cup of coffee a day

Of course, if you're doing any of the things above, you need to stop.

And now let me give you the good news. With my simple cancer-fighting eating plan, you can eat as much and as often as you like as long as you avoid the following five harmful foods:

1. No sugar — in any form. (Stevia and Xylitol are the only sweeteners I recommend for cancer patients.) This is a lifetime commitment, not a temporary measure until you recover.

2. No processed food — in any form. This is the simplest way I can explain what I mean: "If it's not in the form God made it, you don't eat it." Again, this is a lifetime commitment. Processed food is the cause of most major illness. Does this make it difficult to go out to eat — at friends' and relatives' houses or in a restaurant? You bet! Am I saying you need to take your food with you? You bet!

3. No animal protein. Not just red meat but *all* animal protein. Fish, chicken, seafood, shellfish, eggs. Why? Because it's tough for your body to digest. Eating animal protein diverts about 40 percent of your body's energy from fighting the cancer to digesting the protein. Now, when you get rid of your cancer, you can relax this prohibition a little. But *only* a little. One piece of chicken or fish a week, for example. If you don't believe me, please read *The China Study* by T. Colin Campbell, Ph.D. Out of the dozens of books on diet that I've read, this is the only one that gives you *hard science* rather than mere opinion.

4. No dairy. That includes things like milk, ice cream, cheese, and butter. Again, these things are hard to digest and promote cancer. What about my recommendation to eat cottage cheese mixed with flax oil? Remember, I said the cottage cheese loses all its dairy properties when you mix it with the flax oil. It bears repeating that dozens of people I've worked with who are lactose-intolerant can eat the cottage cheese/flax oil mixture with no problems whatsoever. When you're free of cancer, you can relax the dairy prohibition a little, but only a little.

5. No gluten. I'm talking about bread, cereal, and pasta. Some 30 percent of adults are allergic to gluten. Most of them don't even know it because the allergic reaction is frequently delayed for hours or days. But the main problem with gluten is its high glycemic index. That means it turns to glucose rapidly. If you want to feed your cancer cells, eat gluten. Otherwise, avoid it. Most health food stores these days have "gluten-free" crackers and sprouted bread-like products.

What, then, *can* you eat?

No doubt you're wondering what you *can* eat within my cancer-fighting eating plan. Well, the answer is: plenty! Here are some ideas.

1. Lots of raw, whole vegetables. The easiest way to cleanse your entire digestive system and get all the nutrients and fiber you need is to eat *large* salads with a wide variety of raw veggies and a little olive oil and lemon juice on the top — no other salad dressing. What veggies? Dark, green leafy stuff (kale, kohlrabi, spinach, etc.); broccoli; cauliflower; cucumbers; onions (red and yellow); bell peppers (red, yellow and green); radishes; tomatoes; squash; carrots; leeks; sprouts of all kinds; and on and on. Buy "organic" veggies if you can afford them. Steam some vegetables that can't be eaten raw, such as asparagus, green beans, Brussels sprouts, and so on.

2. Sprouted breads of all kinds — English muffins, etc. Just look around the health food store. You'll find lots of gluten-free products. Caution: some of them contain sugar.

3. Preservative-free bread — "Ezekiel" and "Genesis" gluten-free brands are good examples of this kind of bread. You'll find them in the frozen food section of your health food store. These breads have to be kept in the freezer because they have no chemical preservatives. I recommend toasting this bread. You can enjoy it with a little olive oil. No butter, remember?

4. Cereals made with millet, quinoa, etc., and no gluten. Use almond milk on them, not soy milk. (Soy is controversial. Why eat anything controversial when you're sick? Let

others prove who's right.) Just be careful that neither the cereal nor the milk has any artificial or real sweeteners and preservatives.

5. Fruit. Except for the berries or fresh pineapple (another good cancer-fighting fruit) you put in your flax-oil/cottage cheese smoothie in the morning, try to limit your fruit to one piece of whole fruit (apple, banana, handful of grapes, etc.) a day. No fruit juice because it blasts your pancreas with lots of fruit sugar.

What about vegetable juice? Avoid it. Juicers strip vegetables of fiber, and cancer patients need a lot of fiber. You can't afford to be constipated.

Congratulations: You've detoxified your body!

It may not be obvious, but the eating plan I've described above efficiently and thoroughly cleanses and detoxifies your entire digestive system! Eat right, and the junk comes right out of your body! The best and cheapest way to regain your health is to eat right.

You need a state-of-the-art vitamin/mineral supplement — not the drugstore or supermarket kind

The sixth part of my cancer-fighting protocol — what I would do if *I* had cancer — is a state-of-the-art vitamin/mineral supplement. I'm not talking about the cheap, heavily advertised stuff you find in drugstores. Those vitamin/mineral supplements are just about worthless. Indeed, you get what you pay for.

The vitamin/mineral supplement I take and recommend is "Daily Advantage," which Dr. David Williams formulated. This supplement comes in plastic packets, each of which contains eight capsules. I've taken two of these packets a day (the normal dose) for over 10 years, and I attribute my perfect health at age 80 to this product. If you wonder why I recommend it, that's why. It works for me, and I believe it'll work for you, too.

If you find something better, by all means buy it and let me know what it is.

You can get Daily Advantage by calling 800-888-1415 or by logging onto this website: www.DrDavidWilliams.com.

Why you need MORE Vitamin D3

The seventh part of my cancer-fighting protocol is Vitamin D3.

To heal cancer, you have to elevate the Vitamin D level in your blood and keep it high forever. Here's what you need to know in order to get your level of Vitamin D up to where it should be:

- First, assume you're deficient in Vitamin D. Ninety-five percent of the world's population is deficient in it. We don't get enough sun.

- An adequate level of this hormone (it's really not a "vitamin") is essential to recover from cancer.

- To get your blood's Vitamin D to an adequate level, you have to take a high dose (much more than is in the Daily Advantage supplement) for at least five or six weeks.

- An appropriate amount to take immediately is 25,000 I.U. per day in gelcap form.

- As soon as possible, get your Vitamin D level checked. Any doctor can order the simple blood test, which is called the "25 (OH)D" test or the "25 Hydroxy Vitamin D" test. The result will be a number between zero and 100.

- Your results from that first blood test may be in the low 20s or 30s. To recover from cancer, it must be brought up to 70 or higher and maintained there. To raise it to that level usually takes five or six weeks at the elevated dosage above.

- After taking an elevated dosage of Vitamin D for five or six weeks, have your Vitamin D level checked again. If the result comes back at 70 or higher, you can back off to a maintenance dose of 10,000 I.U. per day.

- The only appropriate form of Vitamin D supplementation is Vitamin D3, which is sold over the counter.

- There are many online sources of Vitamin D3, and are all quite inexpensive. The gelcaps come in a 5,000 I.U. and 10,000 I.U. dose per gelcap. Both are available at http://PuritansPride.com. Buy it in gelcap form.

- One last point: Dr. Navarro has warned users of his HCG Urine Test to discontinue taking the Vitamin D3 supplement three days before taking the urine sample. The apparent reason is because Vitamin D3 is actually a hormone and, therefore, can interfere with the HCG Urine Test. More information about Dr. Navarro and his test will be found later in this chapter.

Summary of the seven self-treatments I recommend

Let me give you a summary of my seven-point program that's so concise you can put it on your refrigerator as a daily reminder. These seven things are what you need to do to chase cancer out of your life not just temporarily but for good!

1. Immune-system stimulation — Transfer Point Beta-1, 3D Glucan. One 500mg capsule per 50 pounds (23 kilos) of body weight daily — in the morning, 30 minutes before eating or drinking anything. www.ancient5.com or call 855-877-8220 in Atlanta.

2. Flax oil/cottage cheese "smoothie." One-third of a cup of flaxseed oil mixed with two-thirds of a cup of cottage cheese. Let the mixture sit for five to eight minutes. Then add berries, almonds and walnuts and a little stevia in the blender. Add a little fresh water. Adjust to taste. Blend on the "liquefy" setting. Eat it as soon as it's blended. Order flaxseed oil from Barleans at 800-445-3529 or www.barleans.com. When you've gotten rid of your cancer you can scale back to a maintenance dose, which cuts the amount of flaxseed oil and cottage cheese in half.

3. Heart Plus and Green Tea Extract. Six capsules of Heart Plus (two at a time, three times a day) and three caplets of Green Tea Extract (one caplet three times a day). They should be taken together. The source for both: www.MakingHealthAffordable.com.

4. Barley Power. Twenty tablets per day. Take six or seven about 15 minutes before each meal. If you're not eating three meals a day, take them two hours after eating. Source: Green Supreme, Inc., 800-358-0777 or 724-946-9057 in Pennsylvania or www.GreenSupreme.net.

5. Cancer-fighting diet. Avoid these five foods: sugar in all forms, processed food in all forms, animal protein, dairy (except for cottage cheese/flax oil mixture), and gluten. Maximize raw, whole vegetables. For variety, eat gluten-free, sprouted bread products, flaxseed crackers, cereals (millet, quinoa, etc., without gluten and with almond milk).

6. Vitamin/mineral supplement. Take two packets of Daily Advantage daily. Source: Mountain Home Nutritionals, 800-888-1415 or www.DrDavidWilliams.com.

7. Vitamin D3. Take 25,000 I.U. per day in gelcap form until your blood level tests at the 70 level or higher, which usually takes about five or six weeks. Then back off to 10,000 I.U. per day indefinitely. You can buy the gelcaps from http://PuritansPride.com.

Well, that's it. It's that simple. If you follow this regimen every day for six to eight weeks, you'll not only be healthier, your cancer should

be on the way out. And don't be surprised if you become 100 percent cancer-free.

This simple seven-point program works because it addresses the four characteristics of all cancer that I mentioned at the beginning of this Special Report: 1) it brings more oxygen to the cells, 2) it helps your body change from acidic to alkaline, 3) it detoxifies your body, 4) it boosts your immune system. It also stops the spread of the cancer (metastasis).

My seven-point program will help you knock out cancer like a champ — and to keep it away after you've whipped it.

Best of all, the seven-point program I recommend is surprisingly cheap. During the first six to eight weeks when you're on the full therapeutic dose of the immune system stimulant, the cost will be about $5.15 per day. When you've gotten rid of your cancer, you can go down to a maintenance dose, which will cost about $3.50 per day.

I'm confident everyone can afford that.

The American Cancer Establishment has brainwashed the public that cancer patients need drastic and expensive treatments like surgery, radiation, and chemo — treatments that cost well into six figures!!! If somebody wants those treatments and doesn't mind spending the money, I have no quarrel with their choice. But if I ever had cancer, I'd prefer to get rid of it with gentle, non-toxic treatments that cost only $3 to $5 per day. Doesn't that make more sense?

As I said in earlier chapters, if a dental problem is at the root of your cancer, you must deal with that and solve it. (See chapter two about solving dental problems.) And if an emotional shock or trauma is at the root of your cancer, you must also deal with that and solve it. (See chapter three about resolving emotional issues.)

How can you tell whether you're getting rid of your cancer?

As you use my simple seven-point program, there's an easy way of checking your progress. The results will build your confidence and strengthen your resolve to stay with the program.

I strongly recommend the HCG Urine Cancer Test because it is spot-on accurate, it's inexpensive, and you don't even need a prescription to get it.

HCG stands for *Human Chorionic Gonadotropin*. Knowing that name isn't important. But you might have heard of it in connection with pregnancy tests.

This test looks at abnormally dividing cells. And it tells you the relative number or level of these cells regardless of where they are in your body or where they started. That's obviously a useful fact for cancer patients to know.

The test gives you a single number. If it's 50 or more, you have cancer that requires treatment. If it's zero to 49 you have the normal number of "abnormally dividing cells" (cancer cells) that even healthy people have. The beauty of this test is that it gives you an accurate trend. For example, if you start out at 55, and your next test comes back as 52, you're moving in the right direction. When you hit 49, you can safely schedule your "cancer-free" party.

The test costs only $55. Here's how to prepare your urine sample for the test.

1. From your early morning urine, take 50 cc (1.7 oz.) and add 200 cc (7 oz.) of acetone (available form a hardware store or pharmacy) and 5 cc (.2 oz.) of alcohol, either rubbing or ethyl. Stir and mix well.

2. Let it stand in the refrigerator for six to eight hours until the sediment is formed. Throw off about half of the urine-acetone

mixture without losing any sediment. (Make sure the sediment stays at the bottom of the container. In other words, don't stir it up.) Filter the rest through a coffee filter.

3. When the filtration is over, dry the filter with its sediment. Fold and wrap the filter in a plastic sandwich bag. Send it by regular international Air Mail to the Navarro Medical Clinic, Dr. Efren Navarro, 3553 Sining Street, Morningside Terrace, Santa Mesa, Manila 1016, Philippines. Include a Xeroxed copy of your $55 cashier's check or money order (NOT the actual cashier's check or money order) with the patient's name, address, sex, age, and brief clinical history and/or diagnosis.

Be sure to include your e-mail address so you can get the results the same day your test is processed. Otherwise you'll have to wait for results in the mail. The Navarro Clinic phone number from the U.S. is 011-632-714-7442.

4. Send the $55 cashier's check or money order to Mrs. Erlinda Suarez, 631 Peregrine Drive, Palatine, IL 60067 USA. Mrs. Suarez is related to Dr. Navarro.

Precaution: No sexual contact for 12 days for female patients before collecting the urine sample. For males, no sexual contact for 18-24 hours before collecting the urine sample. **DO NOT REQUEST THE TEST IF THE PATIENT IS PREGNANT.**

For Dr. Navarro's most up-to-date instructions, log onto his website: www.NavarroMedicalClinic.com.

A much easier way to prepare the urine sample, which I highly recommend, is to get the kit developed by one of my readers, Dave Karlovich. Dave's kit is available in both a U.S. format (with the acetone and alcohol you need to prepare the sample) and an international format (without the liquids). The kit includes pictures with step-by-step instructions along with the measuring cups, filters, mailing envelope, customs form, etc. Best of all, one kit is good for *several* of the tests. This inexpensive kit is available at www.JoeBallCompany.com.

Chapter Six
Should you go to an alternative cancer clinic?

Some clients who hire me as a cancer coach get rid of their cancer on their own — without going to any kind of clinic or hospital. Some use a combination of natural and conventional cancer treatments. And some others feel more comfortable using the services of a clinic.

If you're struggling with cancer, do you need an alternative clinic? There's no right or wrong answer to this question. Rather, it's an individual decision. Let me tell you about some of the top clinics.

Dr. Carlos Garcia's Utopia Clinic

One of the top alternative cancer clinics in the world is Dr. Carlos Garcia's Utopia Wellness in Oldsmar, Florida, founded by Dr. Carlos Garcia. He has been helping patients with cancer and other chronic degenerative conditions at Utopia since 2005.

Dr. Garcia's successes in helping patients with deadly cancers heal themselves have made him world famous. People come to him from all parts of the globe. He believes every degenerative disease has a natural, non-synthetic remedy. In fact, Dr. Garcia and I have virtually identical views about what causes cancer and how to overcome it permanently.

Utopia is an out-patient clinic. Patients stay at one of the nearby motels, and the people at Utopia can give you advice about the options for lodging.

I urge you to watch video testimonials from Dr. Garcia's satisfied patients at Dr. Garcia's website www.UtopiaAwaits.com. Look for Candice's testimonial, which is one of the most convincing. Don't miss it! She went through 18 years of suffering and misdiagnosis by 32 doctors before coming to Utopia. Dr. Garcia helped her heal herself by getting the infected cavitations in her jaw cleaned up -- cavitations that had been caused by improper removal of her wisdom teeth. She recovered completely.

For a free consultation about your condition, call Dr. Garcia's office at 727-799-9060.

Dr. John Lubecki's Clinic

Another remarkable doctor I visited is Dr. John Lubecki in Fair Oaks, California, near Sacramento. Dr. Lubecki is an 81-year-old chiropractor with over 40 years of clinical experience. He is an exceptional man!

When my wife and I visited his clinic we were shocked that he devoted eight hours -- from noon to 8:00 p.m. -- introducing us to his healing methods. Throughout the afternoon, he kept saying, "If the world knew what I'm showing you, there would be no more cancer. There is no reason for anyone to be sick."

Dr. Lubecki has a complete diagnostic and treatment system. His homeopathic diagnostic methods identify deficiencies and determine exactly what's needed to correct them. He can also pinpoint the source of inflammation and effectively treat it. For example, he found a serious potential problem in my wife's neck and upper back. He taught her several exercises to correct it. He measured our arterial blood flow and taught us how to improve it. He realigned our heads on the "atlas" vertebrae (the top bone in the spine on which the head rests). This is the only

conventional chiropractic method he uses.

He introduced us to the "soft laser" -- a remarkable $25,000 machine that can heal almost any infection in a matter of minutes. He also showed us how to use the hand-held version of this type of laser at home to treat pain and virtually any other condition.

During the afternoon, my wife and I met a lady from Germany who was there getting her colon cancer healed. She was truly excited about her progress.

I urge you to view the video testimonials on Dr. Lubecki's website: www.Lubecki-Chiropractic.com.

Dr. Simon Yu, M.D.

Now that I've described outstanding clinics on the East and West Coasts, let me tell you about an exceptional clinic in the Midwest. Dr. Simon Yu, M.D., practices medicine in St. Louis, Missouri. If you want to get a good overview of his philosophy and treatments, read his book *Accidental Cure*, available from Amazon.com. I read this amazing book from cover to cover.

Here's a summary of what Dr. Yu has found to be the five principal causes of disease:

- **Parasites** can be eliminated with natural herbs and medication.
- **Toxicity** -- including mercury amalgam dental fillings -- must be removed from the body.
- **Hidden dental infections** must be identified and eradicated.
- **Food allergies** must be identified and resolved.
- **Inadequate nutrition** must be corrected.

Dr. Yu treats people who have consulted with dozens of traditional doctors without getting any relief of their problems. Dealing with the five principle causes of disease is the secret of his success. You'll find many examples and case studies in his book.

To find out more about Dr. Yu's services, including his address and phone number, log onto his website: www.PreventionAndHealing.com.

Calgary Centre for Naturopathic Medicine

Now that I've told you about three clinics in different regions of the U.S., let me tell you about a Canadian clinic I recommend without reservation.

In October of 2010 my wife and I visited a remarkable clinic in Calgary, Alberta. By the end of our visit, we agreed that the two young naturopathic doctors we met are among the most competent medical professionals in the world. My wife was a registered nurse in Spain for 24 years. She knows good doctors when she sees them.

Dr. Jeoff Drobot, N.D., and his partner, Dr. Shaun Riddle, N.D., complained to my wife and me that "we have no model for what we're doing." Well, after seeing what they're doing, we concluded that they ARE the model!

These two doctors have travelled the world, seeking out the best medical minds and finding out about the cancer treatments that really work. For example, they spent a week in Switzerland, consulting the doctors at the legendary Paracelsus cancer clinic. They also visited the top cancer doctors in Germany, picking their brains and studying their equipment. They traveled to the Baltic Sea to spend time with the inventor of a particular electro-medicine device they were interested in. And they spent three days with Dr. John Lubecki. In addition, they've visited the top clinics in Mexico and Central America.

As a result, the diagnostic tools at the Calgary Centre are second to none. After

pinpointing the patient's weaknesses, deficiencies, and problems, they devise effective treatments. These treatments include IVs, injections, blood cleansing, lasers, tailored homeopathic remedies, several types of electro-medicine, supplements, and natural medications.

When you go through the diagnostic process at the Calgary Centre, you'll be astonished to see the amount of health information you get. It will be like a road map to attain optimal health.

Here's the Calgary Centre's website: www.CalgaryNaturopathic.com.

To give you more encouragement that cancer can be healed, let me tell you the stories of a few of the patients who've been in touch with me.

American doctors could learn from Mexican and German cancer doctors

Most American cancer patients don't consider getting medical treatment in Mexico because they assume medical care in America is better. In some ways, American medicine is advanced, but the typical American methods of cancer treatment lag behind those in countries like Mexico and Germany.

America's cancer doctors, with few exceptions, have an abysmal record. You can judge their work by their track record of failure.

As for Mexican cancer doctors, many of them have advanced far ahead of their American counterparts. Mexican cancer doctors can use effective and gentle treatments that are illegal in America, including intravenous Laetrile. What's more, they can practice medicine without being hassled or shut down by their government — as long as they maintain high standards. Mexico has a lot more health care freedom than America.

Marion D. of Pennsylvania never imagined that she would go to a Mexican cancer clinic. At the age of 65, she was diagnosed with severe ovarian cancer in October of 2003. She underwent the customary American treatments for cancer, including a drastic eight-hour surgery.

The cancer had a big impact on Marion's life because she had always been super active. The surgery was devastating not just for her but also for her daughter, Sherri, who cried for a week.

Determined to help her mother, Sherri did some research on the Internet, but everything she came across was bleak. Then Sherri's husband went online and found some encouraging stories about people who beat cancer with gentle, non-toxic methods. He told Sherri, "You just haven't been looking at the right websites."

One of the websites Sherri's husband came across was mine. When Sherri read my book *Cancer-Free: Your Guide to Gentle, Non-toxic Healing*, she says it gave her a whole new perspective. It gave her a feeling of empowerment. She realized you could actually do something to get rid of cancer. You're not at the mercy of doctors.

Sherri says that my book changed her world. She immersed herself in my book and stepped forward as her mother's Number One advocate.

And so Sherri told her mother all about my book, saying, "Look, Mom, if it were me and I had cancer, I'd go 100 percent alternative." But her mother was reluctant to go against *everything* the doctors said. Furthermore, she was already scheduled to begin chemotherapy in a month.

When Marion made her decision, she told Sherri that she couldn't go 100 percent alternative and that she was going to go

through chemo. But she told her daughter, "I'll meet you halfway. I'll do your nutritional program and take the supplements."

That's all Sherri needed to hear. She put together a plan for her mother, based on my book, including the Budwig protocol, boosting the immune system, changing her diet, taking greens and enzymes, changing her body chemistry from acidic to alkaline, eliminating coffee, and so on.

Sherri told me, "You've never seen anybody go through chemo with hardly any side effects. She refused all of the anti-nausea drugs, but she never threw up. And she had so much energy that she was able to keep on working. Because of the program you recommend, my Mom got through chemo like a champ!"

For the next three years, the doctors gave Marion chemo, on and off. And she was able to work full-time even while taking full-blast chemotherapy. She'd take the chemo on Friday afternoon and be back at work on Monday morning.

By 2007, her doctors wanted to put her back on the full program of chemotherapy because a tumor had grown back. Even though Marion had gone through chemo with little difficulty, she was getting weary of it. And the chemo always caused hair loss.

What's more, she was also starting to lose confidence in the therapeutic value of chemo. She began to believe that the alternative therapies were doing more for her than the chemo.

And so Marion told her daughter, "I have an idea about this upcoming chemo treatment. I don't want to do chemo again. I'm ready to do it your way." And Marion also expressed a willingness to undergo treatment at an alternative cancer clinic in Mexico or Germany if necessary.

Tijuana's tumor terminator saves Pennsylvania woman

When Sherri called me for advice about the best foreign clinics, I referred her to my friend and colleague Frank Cousineau, who's more familiar with the Mexican cancer clinics than I am. Sherri read Frank's groundbreaking book *Cancer Defeated! How Rich and Poor Alike Get Well in Foreign Clinics*. (For information about this remarkable Special Report, which has been renamed *Adios, Cancer!*, see www.adios-cancer.com.) After reading Frank's Special Report and speaking to him, Sherri picked Geronimo Rubio, M.D., of the American Metabolic Institute, Hospital San Martin, in Tijuana.

Immuno-therapy is Dr. Rubio's specialty. Dr. Rubio is known as "Tijuana's tumor terminator". Sherri describes him as "passionate" about what he does.

Sherri and Marion went to Tijuana and checked into Dr. Rubio's hospital. Sherri had to get an international cell phone to keep in touch with her office and her financial planning clients while she stayed with her mother.

In addition to a state-of-the-art laboratory and medical equipment, Dr. Rubio's hospital has a bonus for his patients and for those who accompany them: an ozone-purified swimming pool amidst the palm trees in the Mexican sunshine.

Dr. Rubio terminated Marion's tumor with a combination of natural and conventional therapies including *low-dose* radiation and insulin potentiation therapy (IPT), a technique for rendering chemotherapy much more effective.

IPT is a remarkably clever therapy that tricks the cancer cells into letting down their guard so they can be killed off. IPT uses the cancer cells' craving for sugar to destroy them.

Using insulin, the doctor first starves the cancer cells of sugar. And when the cancer cells' sugar craving reaches a peak, the doctor lets them have some sugar — along with a *low dose* of chemotherapy.

IPT has a devastating effect on cancer cells without weakening healthy cells. And the low-dose of chemotherapy causes none of the problems of American-style high-dose chemo. Not even hair loss.

Marion had no hair loss whatsoever from IPT with low-dose chemo at Dr. Rubio's hospital — *none*!

With Dr. Rubio's help, Marion got rid of her cancer. And she's looking forward to her next follow-up visit in Tijuana.

Sherri recognizes that one reason her mother's cancer came back is because she went off the eating plan I recommend for five or six months. Big mistake! Backsliding into old habits made her mother's body chemistry turn acidic again. Her mother is now committed to staying on the eating plan, including the Budwig protocol, to keep her body chemistry alkaline.

Here's what Sherri told me about what it takes to whip cancer:

"Alternative methods are the answer! The way cancer is treated in America is archaic and barbaric. It's all about money and not about healing. It's not the doctors' fault. They were put through the system."

Sherri acted as her mother's advocate during her struggle against cancer. Sherri says, "Having an advocate is the key to healing from cancer. If you want healing and if you want to have a good quality of life, you need to be in the alternative world. Mom has a great, great life. And I absolutely believe she wouldn't have had that life. She'd be dead by now. There's no question about that."

Over the last few years Sherri has helped many others defeat cancer. Her loved ones and friends often turn to her for health advice.

In conclusion, Sherri told me, "You've changed my life and my Mom's life. The experience has been awesome for us."

Dr. Rubio's website is www.RubioCancerCenter.com.

South Carolina woman amazes her doctor

In 2005, 69-year-old Alla from South Carolina learned she had colon cancer in addition to other health problems. Besides having cancer, Alla needed kidney dialysis. Furthermore, she was diabetic, so she was really facing an uphill fight. She underwent surgery, radiation, and chemo, which caused her hair to fall out.

After those treatments, Alla considered herself "cured." She was so certain she was through with cancer that she donated her wig to the chemotherapy department.

But a year-and-a-half later her cancer snuck back, causing Alla to say: "Dang! Now I'll have to buy another wig." She did chemo again until the spring of 2007. The doctors had bad news for her: "Get your affairs in order. There's nothing more that can be done for you."

Sword of Damocles was hanging over her head

Alla's daughter, Cathy, had been trying to persuade her to consider alternatives to the standard cancer treatments. Cathy told her, "*Now* are you ready to listen? *Now* are you willing to try something else?"

A death sentence was hanging over Alla's head like the Sword of Damocles. At least that's what her doctors said. So she had nothing to lose by trying something new.

Cathy convinced her mother to change

to a healthy eating plan, such as I describe in chapter five of this Special Report. All she asked of her mother was a 100 percent commitment and cooperation to the new plan: no cheating! Alla agreed. Cathy read my book *Cancer-Free: Your Guide to Gentle, Non-toxic Healing* and helped her mother apply the treatment regimen I recommend.

Alla went along with the program for six weeks. She considered the flax oil/cottage cheese mixture "the Sherman," meaning that it was as powerful as a Sherman tank in her battle against cancer.

Astonished doctor told her, "Keep doing what you're doing"

At her next follow-up visit, the doctor was amazed and told Cathy, "Hmmm. The last time I examined your mother she had a tumor the size of a potato under her rib. Now it's small." Alla knew the alternative program was working.

The doctor was so impressed, he told Alla, "Keep doing what you're doing."

Although Alla was beating her cancer, she was losing her health battle on the kidney dialysis front. After kidney dialysis she always came home shivering. She was cold all the time. She couldn't live without dialysis. But she hated it and found it intolerable. So she gave up.

She told her doctor, "I don't want to do dialysis any more." He replied, "Without dialysis, you'll last 10 days." And within 10 days she was dead — not from cancer but from kidney disease.

But keep reading! Alla didn't die in vain. What her daughter, Cathy, had discovered about healing from cancer saved another life.

Doctor says, "What's going on? Her cancer is melting away"

One day in early 2008 Cathy bumped into a casual acquaintance named Peggy. When Peggy mentioned that her 80-year-old mother, Beulah, was dying of lung cancer, Cathy immediately sprang into action. She grabbed a copy of my book *Cancer-Free: Your Guide to Gentle, Non-toxic Healing*. Handing it to Peggy, she said, "I don't know what you think about this, but it's not a joke. Turn to the chapter about the diet, and read the rest later."

On March 10, 2008, a doctor had given Peggy's mother Beulah a death sentence, telling her, "We have no treatment for you. You have six months to live." The doctor made it crystal clear that there was no hope whatsoever.

Beulah calmly told the doctor, "The good Lord is going to heal me." She had faith.

When I interviewed Peggy by phone, she told me, "I couldn't put your book down." After reading it, she bought some fresh flax oil and cottage cheese and started Beulah on the Budwig protocol. Beulah also got on my healthy eating plan and later added Essiac tea to her regimen.

You may recall that I mentioned Essiac tea in an earlier chapter of this Special Report. Essiac tea is a traditional American Indian herbal remedy for cancer. Beulah recommends the brand of Essiac brewed by Ginny Darby-Evans. It's called "Just Tea," and you can order it from this website: www.just-t.com. Ginny's store is located at 449 S. Hickory Valley Rd., Sparta, TN 38585. You can also order "Just Tea" by calling (931) 946-7002.

About two weeks after getting my book from Cathy, Peggy called her with some exciting news: "The cancer doesn't seem to be spreading." When Beulah's doctor saw the

improvement, he started pushing for chemo to "knock it out." But Beulah was determined to get rid of her cancer the natural, non-toxic way.

And with each subsequent visit, Beulah's cancer kept shrinking and shrinking. The doctor kept on pushing his chemo, and Beulah kept on refusing it.

The doctor was puzzled. He became unnerved! In exasperation, he wrote in Beulah's chart that she "chose not to have any treatment." But that wasn't true. Apparently the doctor forgot that he had told Beulah in March, "We have no treatment for you." That was the reason Beulah turned to alternative treatments.

Beulah was pleased to find natural health practitioner Penny Mill of Mount Pleasant, South Carolina. Penny gave Beulah electro-dermal screening, a sophisticated method of identifying health problems. (Penny Mill's website is www.healthforlifeinc.com.

During a follow-up examination with Beulah's regular doctor in May, he told Peggy, "I don't know what's going on with your mother, but her cancer is melting away." In June, he couldn't see any cancer on Beulah's x-ray. And in July, he couldn't even find a trace of cancer in her blood. The cancer was gone. So he told Beulah, "You're in remission." Beulah replied, "No, I'm not." He answered, "Yes, you are. When we can't find any cancer, we say it's in remission." But Beulah said, "When God heals you, you're healed." And now that she's committed to a healthy eating plan, she's confident the cancer will never come back.

By Thanksgiving of 2008, the doctor was so astonished that he took Beulah's newest x-ray to the doctor who had taken the first x-ray of her cancer in March of that same year. The doctor remarked, "This can't be the same woman. There's no cancer here!" But it *was* the same woman. She was supposed to have died by September, according to his six-month prediction, but she had made it to Thanksgiving. And she was totally, 100 percent rid of her cancer.

Furthermore, Beulah regained her health without surgery, radiation, or chemo. She's in fine health. Peggy says, "I'm amazed when I look at my Mom."

Peggy loves to encourage people and help them get rid of their cancer. She told me I should list her phone number and e-mail address in case any of my readers would like to contact her. Her phone number is 864-947-9672, and her e-mail address is pdlower45@aol.com.

My clients routinely get rid of cancer using the same natural methods that Peggy's mother used. Shouldn't that be front-page news? Shouldn't this story be on the evening news broadcasts of the national networks? Why does the cancer treatment industry keep these alternative treatments secret?

If the cancer treatment industry is trying to perpetuate a conspiracy of silence, then it's up to people like you and me to spread the truth far and wide. That's the only way to break this conspiracy.

Getting rid of cancer the ancient Chinese way

Mariah P. was nearly 40 years old when she was diagnosed with a rare and deadly kind of ovarian cancer in 1996. She underwent surgery to remove the cancer and one ovary.

In 2005, when the cancer came back, her doctors pushed for a pan hysterectomy. In other words, they wanted to take out her uterus, fallopian tubes, and her last remaining ovary. Mariah said no to that. But she compromised because of pressure from her family and agreed to laparoscopic removal of the tumor.

In March of 2007 Mariah had more trouble with cancer. By this time it had spread to the liver, and her doctor said, "You have three months to live." He recommended chemotherapy. And to this day Mariah believes she would have been dead in three months if she had taken that doctor's chemotherapy.

The doctor only gave Mariah "three months to live." She proved him wrong.

Mariah did some research and found out that chemo wasn't effective for her kind of cancer. She got a second opinion from the Mayo Clinic, which recommended major surgery.

Instead of undergoing surgery or taking chemo, Mariah found a remarkable Chinese healer, Zhengang Guo, M.D., from a unique background. Dr. Guo studied medicine in China and became an oncologist and a surgeon. He also mastered Chinese herbal medicine and acupuncture.

When Dr. Guo came to America he accepted a position at the M.D. Anderson Cancer Center in Houston. M.D. Anderson, which is connected to the University of Texas, is considered the leading cancer hospital in the South. But like other American cancer hospitals, it heavily emphasizes the Big Three: surgery, radiation, and chemotherapy – in other words, cut/burn/poison.

Dr. Guo parted ways with M.D. Anderson and established his own clinic in Chicago. Instead of cut/burn/poison, he offers traditional Chinese herbs, acupuncture, and Chinese massage. He helped Mariah get rid of her cancer using these traditional Chinese therapies. He encouraged her with soothing words: "You are healthy! Hang in there." (The phone numbers for Dr. Guo's three Chicago-area offices are: 312-842-2775, 630-789-2350, and 847-770-6295.)

Mariah believes her cancer stemmed in part from emotional issues. Many of my cancer-coaching clients resolve their emotional issues on their own, with the help of a book such as *The Emotion Code* by Dr. Bradley B. Nelson. But some, like Mariah, prefer to work with a practitioner.

To resolve the emotional issues at the root of her cancer, in the fall of 2008 Mariah sought the help of Christopher Lowthert, D.C., of the Schuylkill Chiropractic Center in Schuylkill Haven, Pennsylvania. Dr. Lowthert practices German New Medicine, a counseling technique that helps cancer patients identify and resolve emotional traumas at the root of their cancer.

Mariah says, "German New Medicine plus Chinese medicine has helped me understand how healthy I am. Cancer isn't as fearful as I once thought. We have to look at our emotional conflicts, change the way we eat, and handle our stress levels. *Stay away from Western medical practitioners as much as possible.*

"Until last fall I was motivated by fear. Now I'm motivated by joy, the joy of life, and living and knowing that the body has amazing powers to heal. People think that when you're diagnosed with the 'Big C' you've got one foot in the grave. I'm living proof that that's not true."

Mariah is cancer-free. She's confident that her future is bright.

Allison's doctor went ballistic!

Cancer made a big mistake when it took up residence in the body of Allison H. of Alberta, Canada. It didn't stand a chance.

Allison's doctor made the diagnosis in June of 2007: breast cancer. She told the doctor, "The lump appeared instantly. I felt it in the shower. One day it wasn't there. The

next day it was." The doctor replied, "That's impossible." She answered, "I don't give a sh*t what's impossible. I'm telling you what happened!"

Her doctor went ballistic. Allison told him, "You know, you seem a helluva lot more upset about this than I am."

When the doctor said surgery was necessary, Allison's husband chimed in, saying, "You've got to do whatever the doctor says!" Allison told her husband, "Oh, shut up! It's *my* health that's on the line. Let's investigate the alternatives."

Allison takes cancer doctors to task for terrorizing breast cancer patients, especially young women with children. For example, when she met with a surgeon, he told her, "You've got six months to live." Most patients would have panicked at those words. But it never entered Allison's mind that she would die of cancer. Still, it makes her angry that any doctor would tell a patient she has only six months to live.

She says, "Doctors shouldn't panic their cancer patients. They should tell them to have faith."

The surgeon gave Allison a choice between a total mastectomy and a lumpectomy with radiation. She asked the surgeon some pointed questions, causing him to say, "I'm starting to feel very uncomfortable in the way you're speaking to me." Her husband explained to him, "That's the way she always speaks."

The surgeon made it crystal clear that the radiation was *mandatory*. He told Allison, "If you don't agree to radiation, I won't do the surgery!" Under duress, she agreed to schedule the surgery.

She was mad enough to slug her doctor!

But Allison says the surgeon really "p*ssed me off." She got so hot under the collar that she knew she had to get out of there "because I probably would've slugged him and gone to jail for assault. When I left I was mad enough to put my fist through the car window!"

After she left, she told her husband, "Nobody's touching me! I don't care if I die of cancer. I'd rather die than submit to their miserable treatments!"

By the next day, Allison had cooled off. She calmly called the surgeon's office and said, "Would you please inform the doctor that I've decided to cancel the surgery because I don't want him to be upset with the way I speak."

She didn't want to be bugged by doctors asking her why she wasn't following up with radiation. As Allison says, "Why the hell should I have radiation when the damned cancer is shrinking without it?"

Allison believes mammograms and biopsies are part of the cancer treatment racket. She says, "All you need is ultrasound. Ultrasounds are cheap."

For breast cancer, she says, "Take your vitamin C — five to 10 grams. Don't let them tell you otherwise. Sunscreens cause cancer. The body needs sunshine, vitamin D, and iodine. We don't get iodine in anything anymore. Take a few drops a day." She also recommends eating lots of raw organic vegetables.

Allison's weakness for candy was tough to overcome. But she overcame it because she learned that sugar feeds cancer.

When her husband started investigating alternative vs. conventional cancer treatments, the truth hit him like a ton of bricks. He could see that conventional cancer

treatments were a racket. And he also saw the conspiracy of silence about more effective natural treatments — a conspiracy that keeps big money flowing into the bank accounts of the chemotherapy drug companies.

Allison says her husband is now "one of the strongest advocates for alternative medicine and health freedom you'll ever meet."

Cancer docs who won't let their loved ones undergo chemo!

One thing that shocked Allison and her husband was the hypocrisy of the cancer treatment industry. For example, a recent survey of the 64 oncologists on the staff at McGill Cancer Therapy Center in Montreal found that 58 of them (91 percent) would *not* take chemotherapy or allow their family members to take it for cancer treatment. Why not? Too toxic and ineffective.

Yet cancer patients routinely get high doses of super-expensive chemotherapy drugs — some costing $10,000 a month or more!

Allison says it's time to stop this medical insanity. She says, "Nobody's screaming loudly enough to these doctors: '*What the hell do you think you're doing?*'" And as a result, too many cancer patients suffer a miserable, ugly, disfiguring death. If Allison and her husband hadn't investigated alternatives, she might have undergone disfiguring surgery and other harsh treatments.

Regarding the breast cancer walks and other fundraisers, Allison says, "They aren't doing anything. All they're doing is repeating yesterday's failed treatments. They're perpetuating cut/burn/poison. And that's insane. The very mark of insanity is doing the same thing over and over while expecting a different result. If you spend 40 hours on the Internet, you'll know as much as any oncologist does."

When Allison told her adult son about her alternative cancer treatment, he said, "Oh, mother. You must have the stupidest cancer on the face of the earth. It'd have to be stupid to invade your body. It doesn't stand a chance!"

A mouse that sneaks into a house full of starving cats would have a better chance at survival than Allison's cancer.

Allison talks to anybody and everybody about alternative cancer treatments. And as a result of Allison's health freedom advocacy, quite a few cancer patients are using kinder, gentler treatments to get rid of their cancer.

Mexican Cancer Clinics

To find out more about the remarkable cancer clinics in Mexico, I recommend you log onto www.Adios-Cancer.com. There you'll find an e-book or a printed version called *Adios, Cancer!* by Frank Cousineau with Andrew Scholberg.

Frank is definitely the world's leading authority on these clinics, having led tours of these clinics for 35 years. In his book, Frank tells you everything you need to know about seven of the clinics. He also tells you where to stay if you're an outpatient, about how much it costs, and even how to get insurance coverage of your treatment. This is by far the best source of information on these clinics.

Frank also gives you his phone number and e-mail address if you want to contact him with questions.

German Cancer Clinics

Andrew Scholberg, the same gentleman who helped Frank Cousineau write the *Adios, Cancer!* book, visited 10 astonishing clinics during his trips to Germany in 2007 and 2010. His e-book about these clinics is outstanding. These clinics use an effective cancer-killing technique used nowhere else in the world: a form of hyperthermia (heat therapy) that uses

short wave radio frequencies to penetrate deep into the body. Healthy cells can handle the heat just fine, but cancer cells can't take the heat!

Andrew mentions many celebrities who have used these clinics to recover. The doctors he interviewed at these clinics have a truly holistic approach to healing.

If I had cancer, I would certainly study this e-book and investigate several of these German clinics. To get the e-book, just log onto this website: www.GermanCancerBreakthrough.com.

Chapter Seven
What is a cancer coach, and do you need one?

Disclaimer:

Although many alternative medical treatments have been successfully used for many years, they are currently not practiced by conventional medicine and are therefore not "approved" and legal (in some States) for medical professionals to prescribe for their patients, although it is legal for individuals to use them at their own discretion. It therefore becomes necessary to include the following disclaimer:

Bill Henderson is STRICTLY an information provider. His coaching service offers information ONLY so that the cancer patient can make informed decisions. The patient must make all decisions about what action to take, and the patient must accept responsibility for any risks involved and is solely responsible for his or her decisions. Bill Henderson offers no guarantees that the patient's decisions will lead to a successful outcome. All responsibility regarding the use of alternative treatments rests with the patient. If you have doubts regarding these things, rely on your conventional doctor.

I recommend that every cancer patient have an advocate. That could be a spouse, an adult child, a brother or sister, or a good friend. In the story about Tijuana's tumor terminator in the previous chapter, Sherri was a wonderful advocate for her mother, Marion. If you have cancer, you need an advocate, period. And maybe that's all you need.

But some cancer patients feel they also need a coach. Whether you need one or not is a personal decision. If you need a coach, you can hire me. I do telephone coaching every day for cancer patients all over the world.

You can sign up for my coaching at the Coaching page of my web site, www.Beating-Cancer-Gently.com/coaching.html. This website tells you how to sign up and how you'll get the most benefit from my coaching services. I charge a one-time fee.

At the web page, you'll have the opportunity to pay the fee using several popular credit cards or PayPal. All I ask is that you read my book *Cancer-Free: Your Guide to Gentle, Non-toxic Healing* (at least Chapter 5 on "Self-Treatments That I Recommend") before you sign up for the coaching. We need to "be on the same page". The book is available at my web site (see below).

If you'd like to listen to the latest information I have on cancer, tune in to my web talk radio show. It's available any time. Each week there is a new, one-hour show with interviews with cancer survivors, doctors and researchers. Just go to this website: www.WebTalkRadio.net. Look on the "Show Hosts" page for "How to Live Cancer-Free" hosted by me, Bill Henderson. If you like, you can download the audio file each week and listen to it on your computer or on a CD in your car.

Wishing you all the best,

Bill Henderson

Author of "Cure Your Cancer" and "Cancer-Free" (Available at www.Beating-Cancer-Gently.com)

Radio host of "How to Live Cancer-Free" (Listen anytime: www.WebTalkRadio.net)